The Pilates Body

The Ultimate At-Home Guide to Strengthening, Lengthening, and Toning Your Body—Without Machines

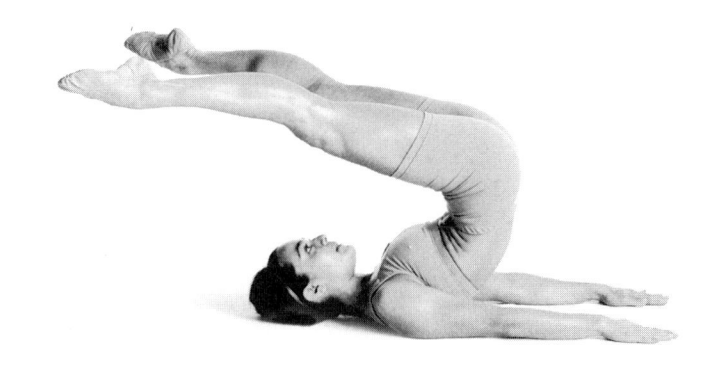

The Pilates Body

BROOKE SILER

Owner of re:AB and Certified Instructor in the Pilates Method®

Broadway Books
New York

BROADWAY

THE PILATES® BODY. Copyright © 2000 by Brooke Siler.
All rights reserved. Printed in the United States of America.
No part of this book may be reproduced or transmitted in any form or
by any means, electronic or mechanical, including photocopying,
recording, or by any information storage and retrieval system,
without written permission from the publisher. For information,
address Broadway Books, a division of Random House, Inc.,
1540 Broadway, New York, NY 10036.

Broadway Books titles may be purchased for business and
promotional use or for special sales. For information, please write to:
Special Markets Department, Random House, Inc., 1540 Broadway,
New York, NY 10036.

BROADWAY BOOKS and its logo, a letter B bisected on the diagonal,
are trademarks of Broadway Books, a division of Random House, Inc.

Visit our Web site at www.broadwaybooks.com

Library of Congress Cataloging-in-Publication Data

Siler, Brooke, 1968–
The pilates body : the ultimate at-home guide to strengthening,
lengthening, and toning your body—without machines /
by Brooke Siler. — 1st ed.
p. cm.
ISBN 0-7679-0396-X
1. Exercise.   2. Physical fitness.   3. Mind and body.   I. Title.
RA781.S5645   2000
613.7'1—dc21   99-36046
CIP

FIRST EDITION

PHOTOGRAPHS BY MARC ROYCE
ILLUSTRATED BY MEREDITH HAMILTON
DESIGNED BY TINA THOMPSON

01   02   19   18

Pilates® and the Pilates Studio® are registered trademarks of Pilates, Inc.,
and are used with permission.

I dedicate this book to the everlasting spirit of my father, Bern Siler, who taught me about the incredible creative power of the mind, the intricacy of the body, and the overwhelming importance of positive thought.

I would also like to dedicate this book to the tireless effort of Romana Kryzanowska to keep alive the spirit of Joseph Pilates and his work. It is through her enthusiasm and integrity for the Pilates method that we all come to benefit.
She is an inspirational example of the powers of devotion and dedication, and it is an honor to continue to study under her.
Thank you, Romana!

Acknowledgments

The author would like to thank the following for their participation in the production of this book:

Photographer extraordinaire: Marc Royce.

Hair, make-up, and style guru: Bryan Marryshow.

Model dynamos: Julianna Womble, Caitlin Cook, and Dana Eisenstein.

To Romana Kryzanowska, Sari Pace, Sean Gallagher, Elyssa Rosenberg and The Pilates Studio for their superb training.

For the use of their clothing: Capezio, Baryshnikov, Danskin, and Norma Kamali.

For their professional support and encouragement: Charles Bergau, Michele Hicks, Kevin Jennings, Erika Morrell, Bruce Lederman, Lauren Marino and the Broadway team, and the entire gang at re:AB. Thank you!

A very special thank you to Debra Goldstein for her never-ending support and enthusiasm! You take literary agenting to a new level!

And to Mom . . . for teaching me that I can do whatever I want to do if I put my mind to it! I love you.

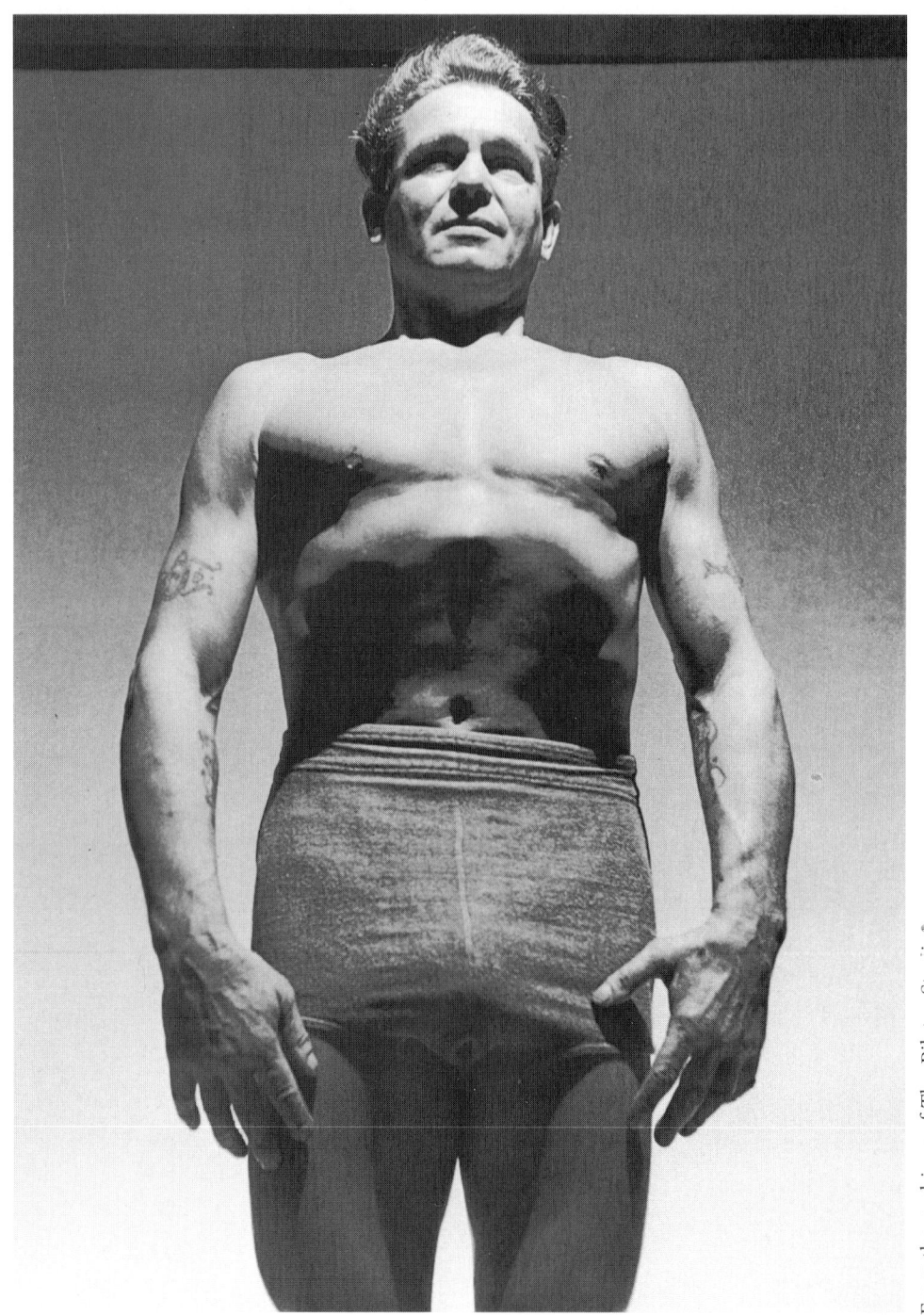

Joseph Pilates, the founder of the Pilates Method of Contrology.

From the archives of The Pilates Stucio®

Physical fitness can neither be achieved by wishful thinking nor outright purchase.

—JOSEPH PILATES

Contents

What Is Pilates?..1
Philosophies Behind the Pilates Method of Body Conditioning..............7
The Matwork Principles..15
Key Elements to Mastering the Mat...19
Frequently Asked Questions..25
The Matwork...33
    Getting Started: Modified Beginner Matwork....................................35
    The Pilates Mat: Full Program..50
    Advanced Extras...145
    The Standing Arm Series..159
    The Wall (Cooldown)..170
The Next Step..174
Glossary...193

What Is Pilates?

The Pilates® method of body conditioning is a unique system of stretching and strengthening exercises developed over ninety years ago by Joseph H. Pilates. It strengthens and tones muscles, improves posture, provides flexibility and balance, unites body and mind, and creates a more streamlined shape.

At a time when the fitness industry is tripping over itself to create new, innovative trends, the Pilates method, with more than nine decades of success, stands out as a tried-and-true formula of wisdom and unwavering results. Pilates was developed to create a healthy body, a healthy mind, and a healthy life, and people are ready to heed its message of balance.

Whether because of a new consciousness or an intense dissatisfaction with the results of trendy exercise programs, in the past five years there has been a tremendous surge in the mind-body focus movement. People are beginning to realize how inefficient the exercises of the 1980s really were. We may have bought into the no-pain-no-gain mentality, but ultimately that led us to spend too much of our precious spare time chained to the gym. We now realize that while exercise should be an important part of our lives, it should add to and not take away from our enjoyment of a full life. With Pilates, specifically the matwork, we can minimize the amount of time spent in a gym or in front of an exercise video, but maximize the results achieved from a full-body workout. The matwork teaches us that the body is the finest and only tool necessary for achieving physical fitness.

Our old exercise regimes are failing us for another reason: They are based on isolating muscles and working each area of the body individually rather than treating the body as the integrated whole it is. The poor physical condition many of us are in today comes from the imbalance of engaging in complicated, inefficient exercises that isolate certain body parts while neglecting others. If our goal in exercising is to balance our bodies, improve circulation, reduce stress, improve endurance, look better, and feel great, then wouldn't it stand to reason that we should utilize the one method that for over nine decades has proven its ability to achieve all these things?

The Pilates philosophy focuses on training the mind and body to work together toward the goal of overall fitness. Although born in a completely different era, Joseph Pilates understood the physical and mental pressures of a busy schedule. He sought to reeducate us to work our bodies with the efficiency of performing our daily tasks in mind. Pilates believed that his method would propel people to become more productive both mentally and physically. For this reason the Pilates matwork is designed to fit into the physical and time constraints of the individual without diminishing its comprehensive elements.

Pilates began developing his exercise system in Germany in the early 1900s. Plagued by asthma and rickets as a child, Pilates' method sprang from his determination to strengthen his frail and sickly body. He called his method "The Art of Contrology," or muscle control, to highlight his unique approach of using the mind to master the muscles. Interned during the First World War, he taught his method to fellow internees and successfully maintained their health through the deadly influenza epidemic of 1918. During the latter part of the war Pilates served as an orderly in a hospital on the Isle of Man, where he began working with nonambulatory patients. He attached springs to the hospital beds to support the patients' ailing limbs while he worked with them, and he and the doctors noticed that the patients were improving faster.

These spring-based exercises became the basis for the apparatus Pilates would later design to be used in conjunction with the matwork. That is why the Pilates name is often associated with antiquated-looking machines, but the matwork is the original movement system that Joseph Pilates created and is just as effective as the work done on the machines. This book shows the entire matwork sequence and has the advantage of being completely portable. The movements of Pilates matwork need no accoutrements and can be performed anywhere a normal human body can fit comfortably when stretched out at full length.

Joseph set up the first official Pilates Studio® in New York City after immigrating to the United States in 1926. Since its introduction to American culture Pilates has maintained a steady and devout following. It has been the secret of dancers and performers since the late 1920s; Martha Graham and George Balanchine were big fans. In recent years it has been discovered by athletes, models, and actors who say they owe their strong, lithe bodies to the Pilates method.

Joseph Pilates authored a book in 1945 called *Return to Life*. That title epitomizes the very nature of the Pilates method. Through concentrated and creative effort you too will reap the myriad benefits that this unique method of conditioning has to offer, reawakening your body through movement and your mind through conscious thought. The combination results in the extra plus of the Pilates method: a revitalization of spirit that is a crucial factor in maintaining good health and a sound mind and body.

"Ideally, our muscles should obey our will. Reasonably, our will should not be dominated by the reflex actions of our muscles." Joseph Pilates believed in the power of our minds to control our bodies. He proved his theory time and again through years of research and training, and his legacy has been passed down through his students.

I have been involved in health clubs in one form or another since the age of fifteen and have tried all that they have to offer. I spent years as a personal trainer using weights and machines and sincerely believed that I had put all the strength into my body that it might need. I was wrong. What I had done was create a bulky, stiff set of muscles in a young, active body. I spent hours in the gym daily trying to create a feeling of well-being that was eluding me at every turn. I continued to have aches and pains that no amount of training would alleviate, and worst of all . . . I was bored!

And then I discovered the Pilates method of body conditioning. Within a matter of weeks I began to feel the internal strength that I had craved. My movements became more controlled and responsive. I was standing straighter and feeling more energized than ever before. After a few short months my bulky muscles began lengthening and my flexibility increased tenfold. I felt as graceful and lithe as a dancer. Subsequently my aches and pains vanished and I found myself enjoying my activities more. Most important, I felt empowered by my newfound knowledge. I was interested. I was in control. I was hooked.

Two and a half months after discovering Pilates I enrolled in the certification course, and in the years since, I have enveloped myself in the world of Pilates as both student and teacher. I have trained for thousands of hours and

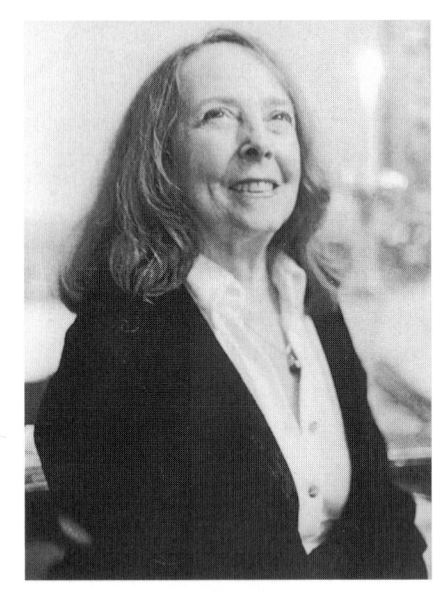

*Master Instructor
Romana Kryzanowska*

have watched the magic of this method unfold before my eyes both in my own work and in the work of my clients.

I continue to study under the master tutelage of Romana Kryzanowska, who was chosen by Joseph and his wife, Clara Pilates, to carry on his work. I bring you *The Pilates Body* in the effort to further expound upon the brilliance of this method in a clear, concise, and creative way. For each movement I have provided visual and verbal cues that will stimulate your mind to action. With patience and perseverance your body will follow, allowing you to experience the efficiency of the Pilates method.

The beauty of Pilates is that once you understand the core of its philosophy, its movements can be translated into any format. Each exercise is an important movement in and of itself and can be used as a way to stretch and move correctly in the course of one's day, but it is not a limited exercise regimen. Many people use the essence of the exercises to enhance other activities; athletes, for example, employ the movements and philosophy of Pilates in their sports. But whether you're an athlete or a couch potato, young and limber or old and inflexible, the Pilates method can and does change the way you relate to your own body and the way you carry it in the world.

The power each of us holds to take control over our own well-being is startling. It begins by becoming aware of our bodies as an integrated part of our creative minds. We were all born with that power. We were all children with active imaginations that continue to live inside us. Sometimes we only need reminding. This book is that reminder. Instead of giving your power away, you will learn to harness it and use it for your very own. This book

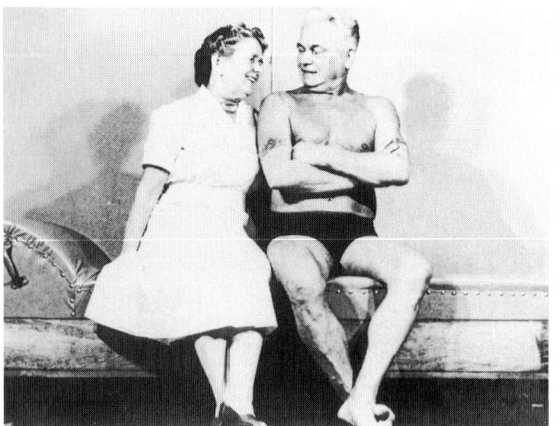

Joseph Pilates and his wife, Clara, on one of the original Pilates apparatus.

From the archives of The Pilates Studio®

will teach you to creatively blend the power of your mind with the movement of your body in a way that is both efficient and extremely enjoyable. It is important that you understand the role you play in all of this. It's all about you. What you put in is what you'll receive, no more and no less.

Remember that with the power of your mind you can bring anything to light, so see your goal and then work to achieve it. This book will serve as a tool to help you along the path, but remember that it is your dedication to yourself that ultimately makes it all possible.

Good luck, and above all else . . . enjoy yourself!

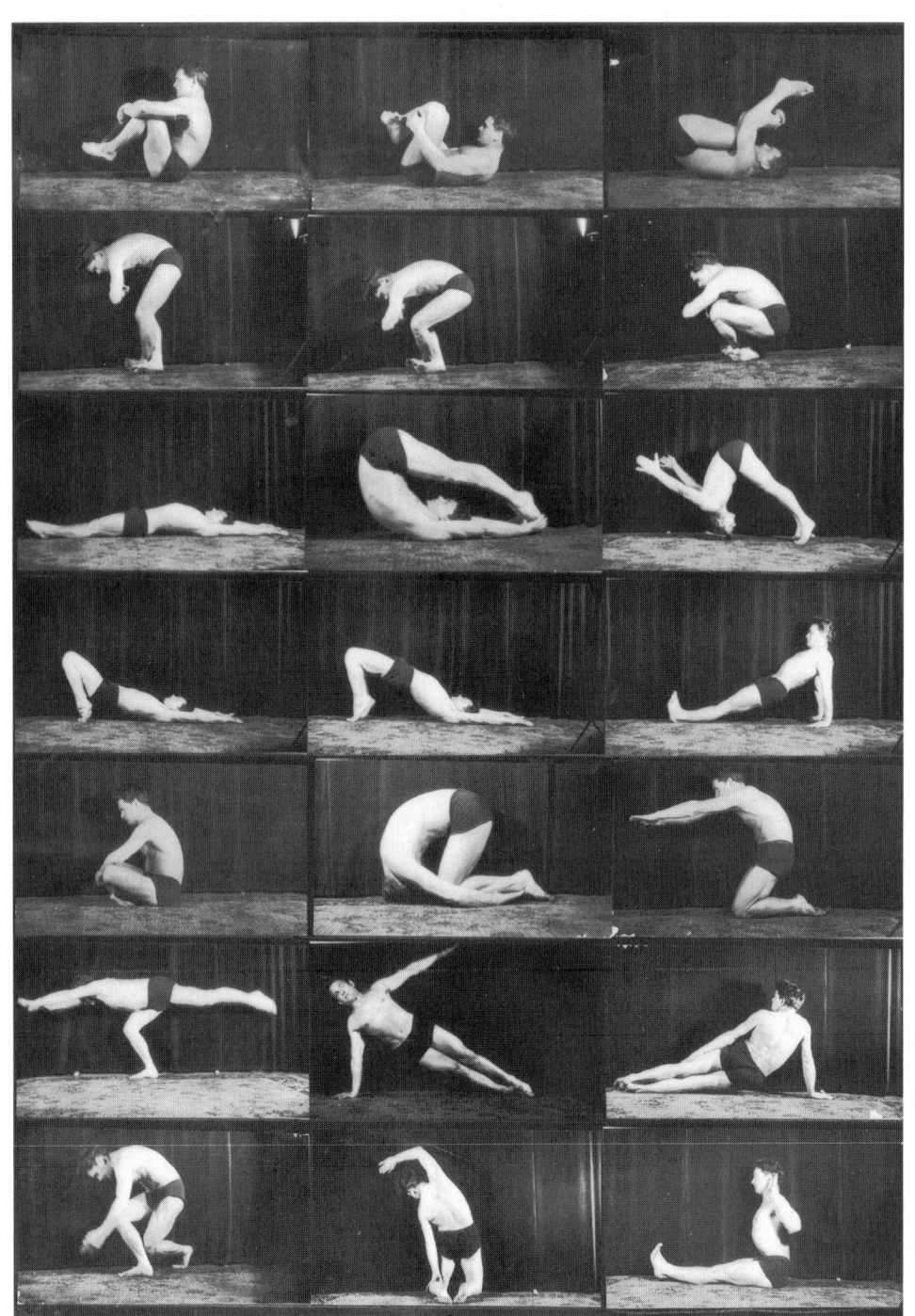

Joseph Pilates demonstrates the "Natural Rejuvination of The Human Body through 'Contrology' Balance of Body and Mind."

From the archives of The Pilates Studio®

Philosophies Behind the Pilates Method of Body Conditioning

"PHYSICAL FITNESS IS THE FIRST REQUISITE OF HAPPINESS"

Joseph Pilates believed that in order to achieve happiness it is imperative to gain mastery of your body. If at the age of thirty you are stiff and out of shape, then you are "old." If at sixty you are supple and strong, then you are "young."

Pilates' development of his method evolved into a vision of an ideal lifestyle, attained only through balance of the physical, mental, and spiritual. Through visualization, physical strengthening and stretching of the body, mental vigor and improved blood flow returns to inactive brain cells. This renewed spirit of thought and movement is the first step toward stress reduction, grace of movement, alacrity, and a greater enjoyment of life.

One of the best examples of this theory is a child at play. The suppleness and vitality of a child are often envied, as if they were traits we no longer possess. Says who? With patience, perseverance, and a strong will all things are possible.

REDUCING STRESS AND FATIGUE

In today's fast-paced life the physical and mental stresses we encounter are dangerous threats to both our health and our happiness. We spend countless hours sitting in front of our computers or bent over our desks, or we're running around, lifting, lugging, and creating havoc in our bodies and minds. Without properly caring for our bodies it is impossible to feel good. Most if not all of our stress and fatigue comes from poor posture, imbalances in the body, and lack of correct breathing. We must first learn to properly strengthen and control our muscles before subjecting them to the rigors of daily living.

These days it seems that only our hobbies and leisure activities keep us relaxed and invigorated, but why should that be so when we can so easily utilize the strength and suppleness inherent in our bodies?

The Pilates method of body conditioning is not an arduous technique that leaves you tired and sore. In fact, quite the opposite is true. By allowing the movements to stretch your body as you simultaneously work on the strengthening elements of the method, you are creating a habit of relaxed effort for your body to follow. We are far too used to straining ourselves in the effort to strengthen our muscles when we should be enjoying the movements themselves.

USING VISUAL IMAGES
TO ENGAGE YOUR MIND AND BODY

Most exercise dropouts claim boredom as their number-one excuse—not hard to believe considering that most people work out only because they feel they "should" and not because it feels good or adds to their mental stimulation.

Think about all the hours you have spent exercising and letting your mind drift away from what you are doing. Instead of watching television or thinking about taxes and baby-sitters, remember what it is you are trying to achieve. Essentially, when you work your body without engaging your mind, you are performing only half a workout. It is the least efficient way to achieve the goals you have set for yourself. The opposite is also true in the lifestyle standards we set for ourselves. By engaging our minds at work without considering the physical toll today's jobs take on our bodies, we are setting ourselves up for a fall. "Sound body, sound mind"—sound advice!

Visual imaging is a relatively new concept in the realm of fitness, but it is by far the most effective. Using visual images to engage the mind is the fastest way to gain access to our complex anatomical system. By using visual metaphors you are able to subconsciously call upon the use of your muscles without needing the technical knowledge of muscles and their functions. If I tell you to "sit up tall as if your head were touching the ceiling," not only are you using your mind's eye to visualize that sensation, but you have also employed myriad muscles you probably never knew existed. You are presenting your mind and body with a challenge that unites their efforts to achieve that goal.

When you create a familiar, albeit imagined, situation within your mind, the body is able to instinctively respond. The creation of that situation is what engages the mind and makes the process more enjoyable. Essentially, it is your own creative ability that will control the actions of your body.

TRIGGERING INSTINCTUAL MUSCLE REACTION THROUGH VISUAL IMAGES

Visual imaging creates a frame of reference for your body to follow. By asking your mind to conjure up images, the innate signaling system of your body is triggered. Like a telephone switchboard, images are routed through your brain and transferred into instinctual movements. Imagine how your body would react if you were punched in the gut. Not pleasant, but the thought alone is enough to trigger a physical response. Similarly, expressions such as "walking on air" or "a spring in your step" can be manifested physically.

The movements of the matwork will become as much second nature as skipping, twisting, reaching, or bending over to pick up a dropped pen. The benefit is that you no longer need to think of movement as belonging only in an exercise class. You will begin to trigger the same awareness in the movements of your daily activities that you have while focused in a class.

Pilates believed that proper movements should become as natural to a person as they are to an animal. When an animal raises itself off the ground, it stretches from its head to its claws to its tail. It leaves nothing out. When we humans move, we tend to focus on one area or another and ignore the rest. The irony is that most everything we do, from walking to sitting up, can and should utilize all our muscles.

Subconscious rhythm is inherent in us all. When we walk, run, gesture, and move in general, we do so without thinking. This is the way it should be, and this is the way the Pilates method was designed to work. By flowing from one movement to the next, you will re-create the natural rhythm of the body. I have made sure to include transitional directions in each exercise so that as you progress you will know how to move smoothly from one exercise to the next.

The goal of the matwork sequence, at any level, is to create a natural flow of movement and then to gradually increase the dynamic, or energy, with which you perform the movements without sacrificing control. Eventually the time it takes to complete your mat sequence should decrease to where you can choose some or all of the exercises and not lose the efficiency with which you perform each one.

MAKING THE CONNECTION BETWEEN PILATES AND YOUR DAILY ACTIVITIES

At first the movements of the matwork may seem unconnected to your daily routine. However, with patience and persistence you will begin to understand how the movements are merely tools to understanding your body. Once learned, muscle control can be applied to any function of physical movement, from walking and running to lifting and carrying.

Structured around the stomach, hips, lower back, and buttocks—the center of the body, or its "powerhouse"—the movements of the Pilates method are instrumental in maintaining good posture and alignment. These are key elements in proper muscle use and make even the most difficult daily tasks seem effortless.

"NEVER DO TEN POUNDS OF EXERCISE FOR A FIVE-POUND MOVEMENT"

If there is one true misconception in exercise, it is the belief that more is more. An attitude such as "This feels like it's really working—let's do a few more sets" is pointless. It's like doubling up on your medication to get better faster. You end up doing more harm than good because you are exhausting your muscles. In a sense, the Pilates method is to exercise what interval training became to aerobics: a more comprehensive way to work your body within the limits of muscular endurance.

The concept of working all the muscles simultaneously but continually switching movements is the most efficient way to build stamina. Because all the muscles of the body are being used simultaneously, and during each and every exercise, there is no need to try to load up on one area.

QUALITY VERSUS QUANTITY

Just because it's not burning doesn't mean it's not working! If I had a nickel for every time I've had to prove that exercise can work without pain, I'd be a very rich woman.

I know that quite a number of exercisers have grown accustomed to the soreness associated with working out and find it rather addictive, but such soreness is not an indication that the workout is actually efficient. Muscle soreness is a direct result of lactic acid buildup in the muscle, improper stretching, or the tearing of muscle tissue. The energy your body needs to expend to repair damage or counteract fatigue is precisely what takes away from the efficiency of the workout.

Pilates was designed to work directly with the deepest muscles in the body, creating a strong core without the pain associated with conventional exercises. And because you stretch your muscles as you strengthen them throughout the sequence of a Pilates workout, there is no fear of being improperly warmed up. There is no ripping of muscle tissue, jarring impact on your joints, or exhaustion of your muscles beyond effectiveness. Each movement has a prescribed maximum number of repetitions. The reason for this is, assuming you are doing the exercise correctly, that you are working your muscles so precisely and efficiently that doing any more is completely unnecessary.

Most exercise techniques focus on the superficial muscles in the body and pump them up for effect. This is fine if bulk is your goal; however, thick, stiff muscles are not necessarily an ideal. For example, the hulking muscle of Arnold Schwarzenegger may be considered attractive by some, but sheer mass inhibits a muscle's ability to move freely. In comparison, the lean and lithe muscles of Bruce Lee are testament to the fact that you can heighten a muscle's efficiency by combining grace of movement with strength.

TAKE BACK YOUR POWER BY BELIEVING YOU CAN

The first and biggest hurdle in exercise is combating the mind's self-deprecation. Many people come to my studio and instinctively begin reciting their shortcomings: "I'm weak," "I'm uncoordinated," "I'm lazy." They are looking to me to fix their bodies, but the truth is that becoming dedicated and succeeding in fitness are already within their control. If you have made the effort to get to an exercise studio or to buy and read this book, then there is already something wonderful stirring inside you. Reward your new desire for change with positive thoughts rather than dwelling on the deficiencies that brought you to this point.

Believing in your innate ability to achieve is the key to changing your body. It is as simple and charming as the age-old tale of *The Little Engine That Could*. While the vast majority of Americans have forgotten this concept or think they have outgrown it, I assure you that it still holds true.

I am lucky in that I get to watch small miracles happen every day. I have watched the weary become strong, the stiff become flexible, and those suffering from pain become pain-free. There is only one reason this happens, and it is because they have come to believe that they can. There is nothing that we cannot achieve if we put our minds to it, and this is especially true when we are speaking about our own bodies. We spend the majority of our lives trying to influence external forces over which we have little or no control, when the very thing over which we have complete control is literally beneath our own noses.

The many clients that I train on a daily basis all have one thing in common: my constant positive bombardment. Their success comes when they begin believing the positive feedback themselves. Real strength begins in the mind. Stop giving your power away. There is no one who should care more about your success than you do!

COMMITTING TO PHYSICAL AND MENTAL SELF-IMPROVEMENT

In Pilates, as well as in life, there is nothing that will work for you that you do not *make* work for you. There is no good fairy who will come to you in the night and transform your body for you. The physical and mental commitment you must make to achieve your goal is the most important step in the process of change.

Believing in and following the Pilates philosophy will be the closest you come to making a miraculous change in the way you look and feel. Take the time to understand the essence of each exercise and to enjoy the freedom of movement, and in time you will create the results you are looking for.

BREAKING AWAY FROM THE GYM/TRAINER TRAP

As strange as it may sound coming from a personal trainer, I do my best to promote self-sufficiency when it comes to exercise. The Pilates method is an education in body awareness and is meant to provide you with the necessary tools for taking care of yourself. If your gym closes early or your trainer is not available, it is not an excuse to sit home and do nothing.

Autonomy is a powerful tool against the risk of failure in exercise. For this reason the Pilates matwork is designed with the intent of making you the master of your own fitness destiny. Whether you do five or forty-five minutes a day, committing yourself to your body is the key.

Pilates at 57   Aug. 1937

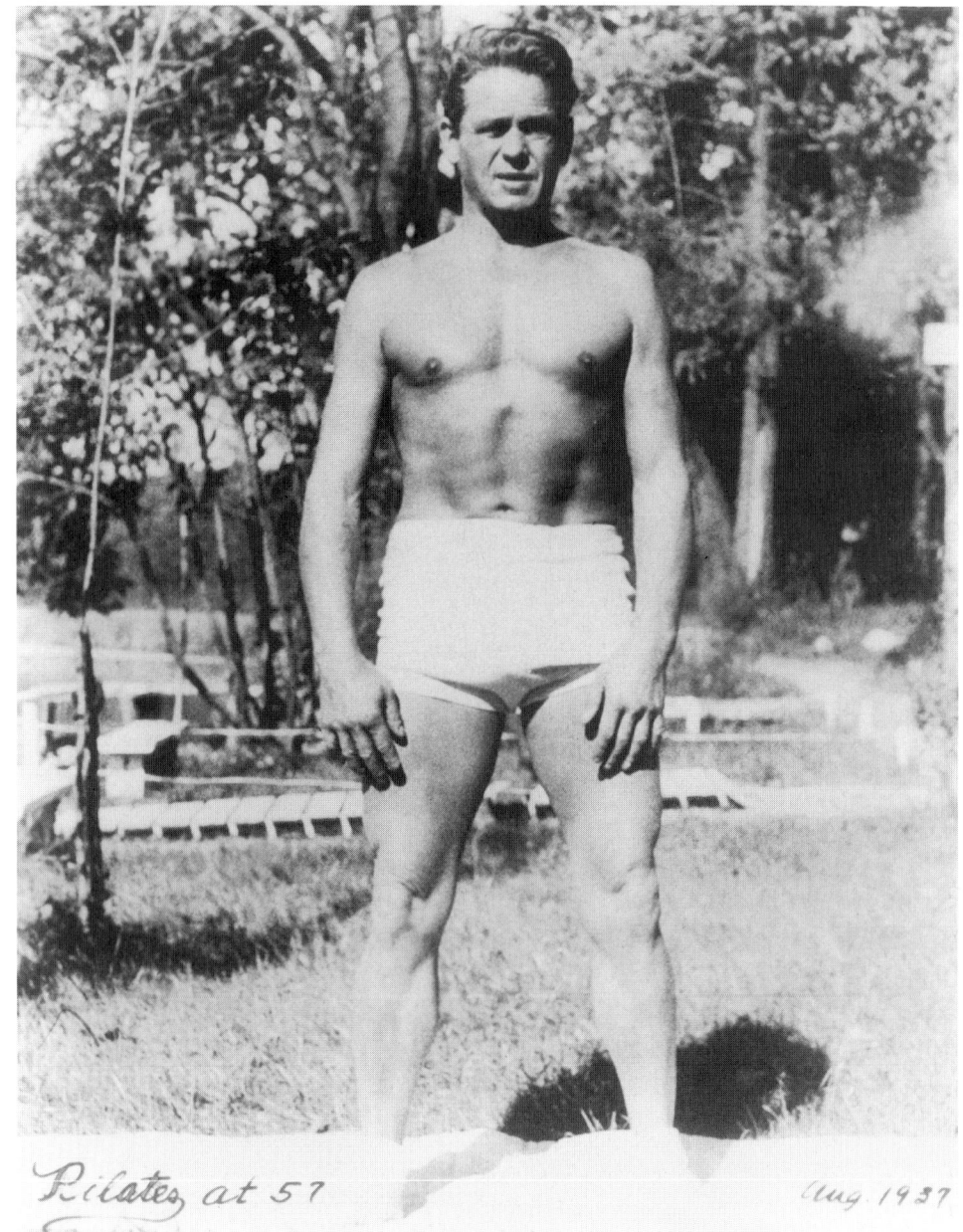

The Matwork Principles

While Pilates draws from many diverse exercise styles running the gamut from Chinese acrobatics to yoga, there are certain inherent ruling principles that bring all these elements together under the Pilates name:

CONCENTRATION

Concentration is the key element to connecting your mind and body. In order to work your body, you must be present with your mind. It is your mind that wills your body into action. Pay attention to the movements you perform and note how your muscles respond to the attention. When you focus on an area, notice how much more you can feel that area working. That's the power of your mind! Use it!

CONTROL

Joseph Pilates built his method on the idea of muscle control. That meant no sloppy, haphazard movements. This is the primary reason injuries occur in other exercise methods. Imagine gymnasts, acrobats, or dancers performing their skills without control. Disastrous! The movements of the matwork are no different. They must be performed with the utmost control to avoid injury and produce positive results. No Pilates exercise is done just for the sake of getting through it. Each movement serves a function, and control is at the core.

CENTER

Think about the muscles you use to go about your daily tasks. For most people it is the arms and legs that get used the most, but what about our center? We have a large group of muscles in our center—encompassing our abdomen, lower back, hips, and buttocks—that are begging for attention. Pilates called this center the "powerhouse." All energy for the Pilates exercises initiates from the powerhouse and flow outward to the extremities. Physical energy is exerted from your center to coordinate your movements. In this way a strong foundation is built upon which we can rely in daily living.

FLUIDITY

Part of the uniqueness of the Pilates method comes from the fluidity with which the exercises are meant to be performed. There are no static, isolated movements because our bodies do not naturally function that way. Dynamic energy replaces the quick, jerky movements of other techniques. A focus on grace of motion is emphasized over speed, and ultimately the movements should feel as fluid as a long stride or a waltz.

PRECISION

Every movement in the Pilates method has a purpose. Every instruction is vitally important to the success of the whole. To leave out any detail is to forsake the intrinsic value of the exercise. Therefore, choose to focus on doing one precise and perfect movement over many halfhearted ones. Eventually, this precision will become second nature to you, and anything less will be just that.

BREATH

Breathing is the first act of life and the last, and so it is imperative to learn to breathe correctly. In order to achieve his ideal of total fitness, Joseph Pilates designed his method to cleanse the bloodstream through oxygenation. By employing full inhalations and full exhalations, you are expelling stale air and noxious gases from the depths of your lungs and replenishing your body with fresh air to energize and revitalize your system. You will find that proper breathing will help to control your movements both during the exercises and in daily life.

Most books on the Pilates method are content to end with the discussion of the previous six principles, which are indeed the foundation of the exercises. However, there are three additional principles that are crucial to the actualization of your exercise goals. Though they are rarely mentioned in today's fitness world, devoted practitioners of the Pilates method and anyone truly dedicated to the pursuit of the mind-body connection understand that employment of these principles is the difference between simply doing the exercises and experiencing them to their fullest.

IMAGINATION

Our minds work in mysterious ways, and one of those ways is our ability to create a visual framework for our bodies to follow. Our minds act as a switchboard through which we can signal instinctive physical response. We can literally spur our bodies to action through an undercurrent of creative thought. In *The Pilates Body* you will use your mind's eye to enhance your physical movement. I have included both visual and verbal metaphors to reinforce the essence of those movements. Be creative!

INTUITION

Listening to our bodies is something we rarely do. We tend to take the power of our natural intuition for granted. Most of us push our bodies through pain, sickness, and exhaustion, often resulting in discomfort and injury. The Pilates method is based upon the ideal of well-being and is not another mind-numbing, quick-fix solution to fitting into a bikini by summer. Do not force what is not natural. If something hurts, stop! As you will be acting as your own guardian and trainer, it is vital that you trust what feels right and what doesn't. In time you will be able to feel the effectiveness of the exercises as you perform them, in turn creating the results you are looking for.

INTEGRATION

Integration is the ability to see your body as a comprehensive whole. Each exercise in the matwork employs every muscle from your fingertips to your toes. In the Pilates method you will never isolate certain muscles and neglect others. The very idea of isolation creates an unbalanced body that impedes flexibility, coordination, and balance. Uniformly developed muscles are the key to good posture, suppleness, and natural grace. Through integration you will learn to use every muscle simultaneously to achieve your goal. Your mind is the coach and the muscles of your body are your team. No one sits on the bench!

Key Elements to Mastering the Mat

In order to gain the most from your mat workouts, it is important to understand the key elements that are in play. There are many concepts within the whole that may require a variation of what you have been taught in the past.

Remember that opening your mind to new information is the first step toward achieving your goals.

1. REDEFINING THE BODY

Classically we have thought of the body as two arms, two legs, a torso, and a head. In the matwork the key to understanding the movements comes from imagining the body in its simplest form: the torso. The torso (see Fig. 1) encompasses the space starting from just beneath the skull and continuing down to the bottom of the buttocks. It contains the vertebral column (spine) and all the major organs. The "powerhouse," from where the exercises initiate, is also contained within the torso. By visualizing the body in this form, it is easier to understand the essence of the exercises. Your arms and legs will certainly be working; however, it is important not to focus on the extraneous parts of the body as much as the muscles radiating from the body's core, or powerhouse.

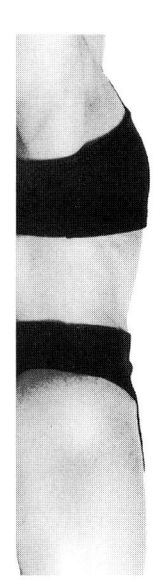

Figure 1

2. YOUR POWERHOUSE

All Pilates exercises initiate from the muscles of the abdominals, lower back, hips, and buttocks (see Fig. 2). The band of muscles that circles the body just under your belt line is termed the "powerhouse." If you think about how you sit and stand, you will probably find that you sink most of your weight into these areas. This not only causes undue stress on the muscles of the lower back, resulting in soreness and promoting poor posture, but also helps create the "gut" and "love handles" that we all strive so hard to combat.

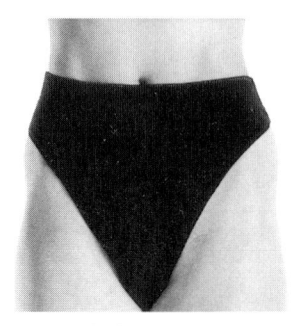

When performing the mat exercises, remember that you should be constantly working from the powerhouse and lifting up and out of this region. Imagine stretching your upper body away from your hips as if you were being cinched in a corset. This action of pulling up and in simultaneously will automatically engage your powerhouse muscles and help protect your lower back.

Figure 2

3. "SCOOPING YOUR BELLY," OR NAVEL TO SPINE

In many exercise methods we are taught to bear down on the abdominal muscles, pushing them outward into a little hill of sorts. The action of this technique builds the muscles outward and tends to push them away from the spinal column. The result of training your muscles in this way is either to develop a slight sway in the lower back that makes it truly difficult to support the lower lumbar region of the back, or to develop a thick middle whereby your back is supported by the mass of contracted muscles that makes having a waistline virtually impossible. When learning the matwork a very different technique is emphasized. You will learn to "scoop" your belly, or press your navel to your spine, thereby using the abdominal muscles to reinforce the paraspinals (muscles that run alongside your spine). This action not only strengthens and stretches the muscles of the lower back considerably but also allows for the creation of a flat abdominal wall. Pressing the navel to the spine is very often confused with sucking in the stomach, but this is not the case at all. By sucking in your stomach you automatically hold your breath, the very antithesis of the desired effect. Instead think of a weight pressing your belly down to your spine, or an anchor attached to your belly button from the inside and pulling it down through the floor (see Fig. 3). Learn

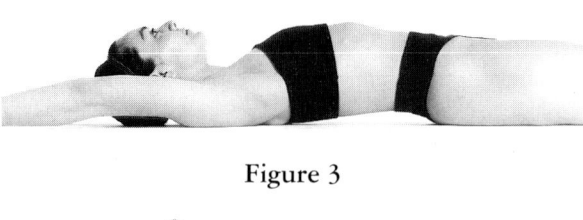

Figure 3

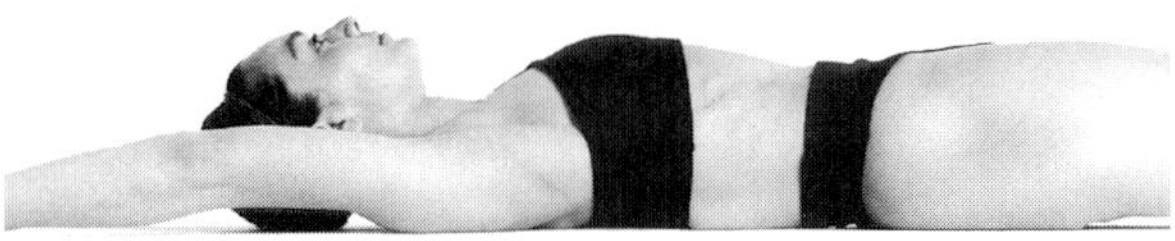

to maintain this feeling while breathing normally, that is, taking in and expelling air from the lungs and not from the belly, as taught in many other techniques.

4. TUCKING UNDER VERSUS LENGTHENING

In Pilates it is key to keep lengthening your muscles as you strengthen them, therefore, any movement that instructs you to "squeeze your buttocks tightly" is not meant to cause you to tuck your bottom under or contract your muscles so strenuously that your bottom curls up off the mat. Ideally, your pelvis and the base of your spine should stay pressed against the mat or be held firmly in position by the surrounding muscles of the powerhouse.

If you are new to Pilates, it may seem difficult for you to begin some of the movements without a slight tuck, and that's okay. Just be aware that your goal is to gain strength and control to be able to lengthen in opposition to your pelvis; in other words, stretch away from it, and keep it stabilized throughout the exercise movements.

5. INTEGRATED ISOLATION

One very important and unique element of the matwork is learning to rethink the point of focus when you perform the movements. It is commonly thought that the areas of the body that are in motion during an exercise are the areas on which the mind should be focused; this is known as "isolating" a particular group of muscles. The problem with this ideology is that it ignores the other areas of the body that are not in motion, creating an unbalanced body. When performing the matwork, however, it is important that every muscle of the body be working simultaneously, since that is the natural inclination of the body and also maintains the body's sense of balance. In order to achieve this goal during the matwork, it is most effective to think of focusing on stabilizing, or anchoring, the area of the body that is *not* in motion. For example, in the Roll-Up (see Fig. 4), by focusing your mind on stabilizing your lower body while your upper body is in motion, the muscles of your entire body are engaged in a symbiotic and highly effective

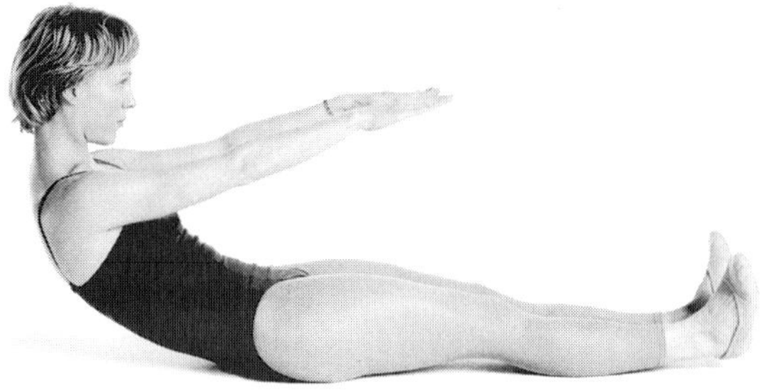

Figure 4

manner. Generally, when you attempt this exercise focusing only on the lifting and forward motion of the upper body without first anchoring and focusing on the lower body, you create a very sloppy and ineffective exercise that can lead to injury.

6. STABILIZATION USING THE PILATES STANCE

Very often in the movement descriptions you will come across the expression "Squeeze the backs of the upper inner thighs"; this action is used to engage and stabilize the lower body. The "back of the upper inner thighs" is meant to express a slight turnout of the legs initiating from the hip joint. This slight movement disengages the quadriceps (thigh muscles) and engages instead the target areas of the hips, buttocks, and outer and inner thighs. Think of turning your thighs to face away from each other and holding a tennis ball between them (see Fig. 5). Your feet should remain in a small V position with the heels glued together. Your knees should remain "soft," straight but not locked.

In the beginning you might find that it is not easy to turn out at the thigh without also turning out the feet, but it is important that you master this position so that you may correctly perform the exercises. You will also find that during the progression of movement of the exercise the legs will want to turn back inward; this is precisely the point at which focusing on the stabilization of the leg position is most important. Continue squeezing the buttocks and backs of the upper inner thighs together and feel the effort created throughout the entire torso as you do so.

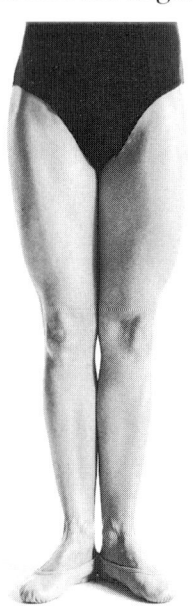

Figure 5

7. MUSCLE CONTROL WITHOUT TENSION

One of the most difficult concepts of the matwork for most people is the idea of engaging and controlling the muscles without tensing. We have become conditioned to tense up, hold our breath, and push to the point of strain in order to achieve our exercise goals. The matwork will serve to dispel those fallacies and retrain you to see the efforts of the movements in a much more natural way.

Think about a dancer as he/she performs; while you know how much strength and effort it takes to perform the complicated dance moves, it often appears effortless and natural. The same principle is at work while performing the mat exercises. While the movements require strength and concentration, there should always be a natural flow and rhythm that serve to relax the muscles without disengaging them from their task. This relaxation needs to begin in the mind and circulate throughout the muscles of the body. Breath is an effective tool for achieving this state. While the breathing should feel natural, inhaling at the beginning of a movement and exhaling throughout its completion, there are times you will find you are holding your breath because the exertion is too great. This defeats the purpose of the exercise. Make sure that (1) you have made the necessary modifications to ensure that you are working at the proper level for your body and, (2) you are not tensing your muscles as you perform the movements. Remember that there is no one testing you. If you begin gradually, mastering the important elements of the movements first, the rest will undoubtedly follow.

Be patient and enjoy the process!

8. MODIFICATIONS FOR THE MOST COMMON PAINS AND INJURIES

No exercise in the Pilates method should cause pain. Ever!

If you find an exercise putting an uncomfortable strain on an area of your body, stop, review the instructions to make sure you are working from the proper muscles, and try again. If you still experience pain, leave that exercise out for now. As your strength and control increase, you will be able to come back to that exercise in time. Remember too that some exercises may not be suited to your individual body. Use your best judgment and listen to your body!

Lower back pain is most often caused by pushing your abdominal muscles away from your back, leaving little support for the muscles of the spine. To combat this habit, focus on pulling the navel to your spine, as if the actual belly button is, in fact, a button that is fastened to your spine. The deeper the stomach "sinks" into your spine, the safer your back will be. When horizontal, imagine a heavy metal plate anchoring your belly to the mat beneath you. When vertical, imagine a rope through your center pulling your belly back.

Knee pain is most often caused by improper foot and leg positioning, or by gripping or overextending the muscles around the knee joint. Try to maintain a "soft" knee while executing the movements and use the muscles of the inner thighs and buttocks to compensate instead. Throughout most of the exercises, and especially while standing, use the Pilates stance to support your weight. (See Figs. 6 and 7.)

Neck pain is most often due to weak muscles or tightening your shoulders to support that weakness. As you perform the movements of the matwork remember to stay lifted using the muscles of your abdominal region and not the neck itself. Always lower your head and rest when you feel you are exerting too much effort from your neck. If needed, you can place a small pillow under your neck for support.

9. LENGTHENING YOUR NECK

It is a common mistake in Pilates to tense up in the shoulders as you perform some of the movements. In order to avoid this bad habit, it is important that you think of lengthening the vertebrae just below the skull by pressing the back of your neck toward the mat when lying flat or pressing out through the crown of your head when sitting, standing, or stretching forward. This adjustment will release the muscles of the neck and shoulders and allow you to focus on your powerhouse instead. Think of bringing your chin closer to your chest to achieve this sensation.

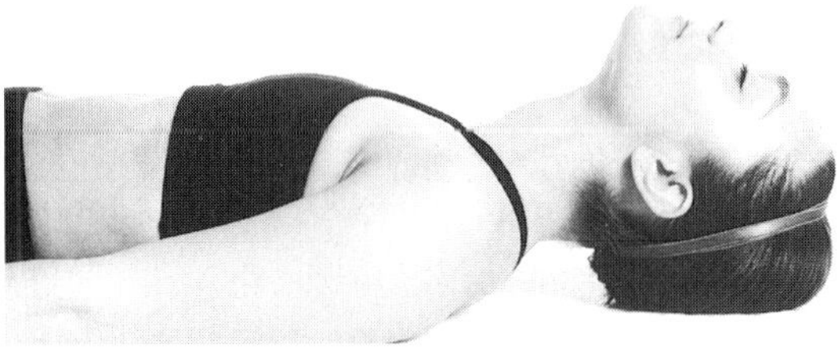

Figure 6

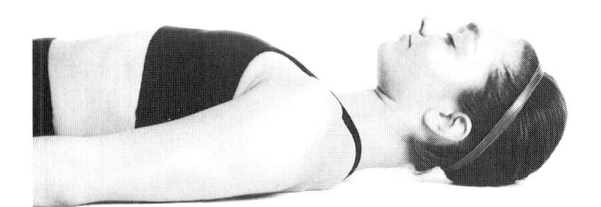

Figure 7

Frequently Asked Questions

WHY THIS FORM OF PILATES?

Over the years Pilates has taken on many different shapes and forms as it has passed from teacher to teacher. Some styles have taken on a genuinely therapeutic approach and are taught in a slower and more deliberate manner. Others have maintained an athletic and more dynamic approach focusing more on movement and rhythm. In its essence Pilates is meant to stretch and strengthen the body in keeping with balance and alignment. Posture, length, and muscle control is at Pilates' core and many different styles of teaching are employed to reach these goals.

There has been much controversy over what can be deemed true Pilates, and in some cases we must agree to disagree. However, Joseph Pilates, in his own books, made it clear that his method was meant to propel us forward to becoming responsible and in control of our bodies and our health. He sought to enlighten, invigorate, and empower us and to that end you must find what works best for you, your lifestyle, and your goals.

Before going into detail about how to use this book to best advantage, I want to address some of the most common questions about the Pilates method.

What is my goal with the matwork?

You are working to re-create your approach to exercise. By using the matwork movements and philosophy, you will create a system that is the most beneficial to your individual body and lifestyle. You are reteaching your body lessons of correct form and movement that will stay with you for a lifetime. Your overall goal is to break bad habits and to connect to and form an alliance

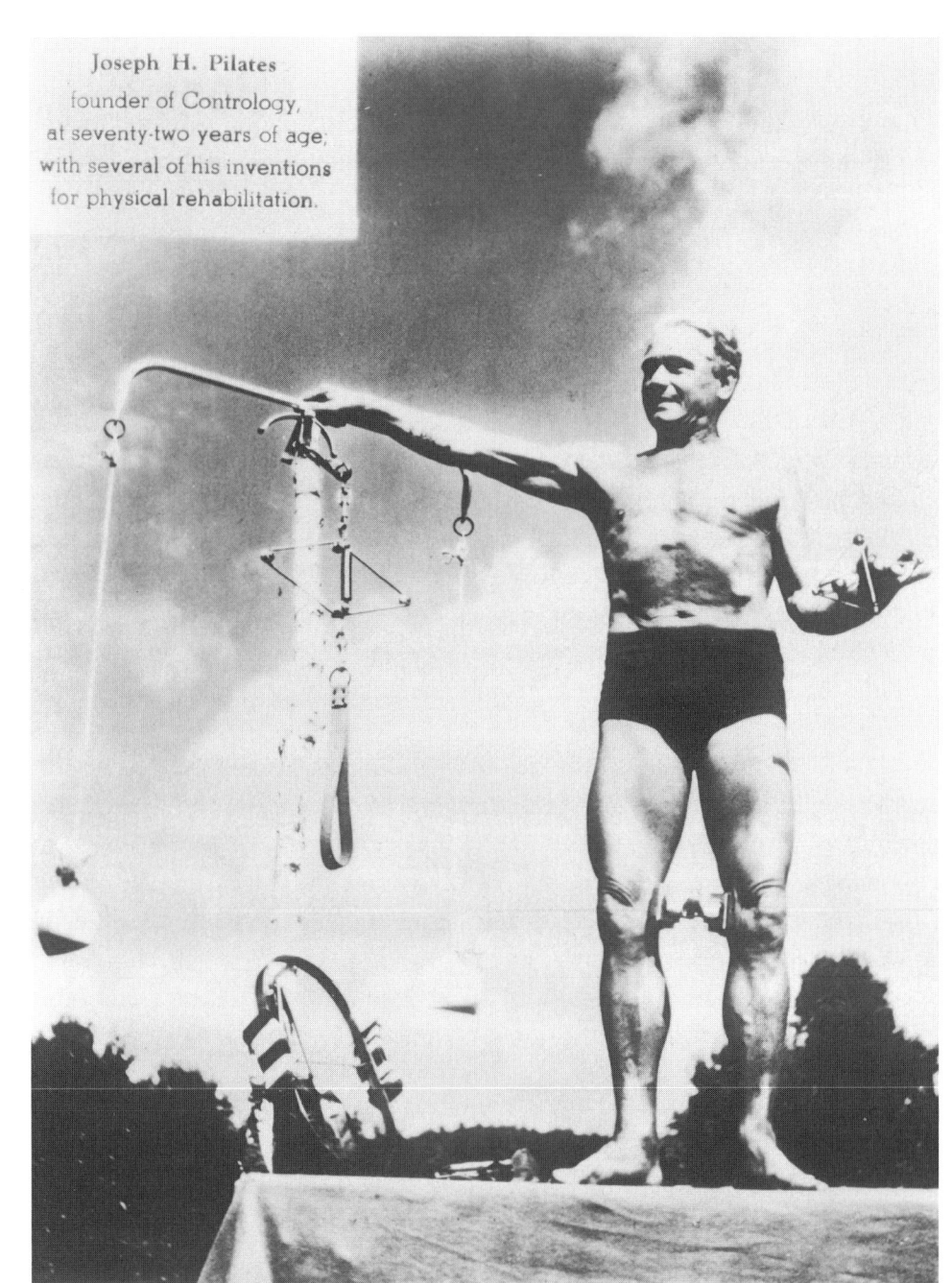

Joseph H. Pilates founder of Contrology, at seventy-two years of age, with several of his inventions for physical rehabilitation.

From the archives of The Pilates Studio®

with your body. For most this means the enjoyment of moving correctly and reaping the benefits of what that brings: better posture, a strong center, suppleness, alacrity, and a feeling of well-being.

Your exercise goal is individual. In the beginning you should aspire simply to master the beginning exercises of the mat (see "Getting Started" on p. 35) by giving your body the chance to perform them regularly. This takes patience and persistence. Don't give up if you can't get all the movements right away. You are working new muscles, and it will take a little time to accustom your body. Even some of the fittest athletes of our time have had difficulty properly performing these movements!

If you are working to advance to the highest matwork level, then your goal is to hone your routine to where you can add new exercises without sacrificing time. This in no way means that you should speed through what you already have learned to get to something new. You want to move with rhythm and dynamic but without surrendering control. Effort and sweat are sure signs that you are accomplishing your goal, but strain and sloppiness are not!

Each and every exercise lends itself to the importance of the whole. Some of the advanced exercises may not be best suited to your particular body. That's okay. Discover what feels best and perfect what you know. Soon you will find that you don't know how you ever lived without it!

Will I be able to do this if I have not been exercising regularly?
As with any exercise program, it is important to check with a physician before beginning. If you are pregnant, injured, or in any way incapacitated, it is imperative that you get the approval of your doctor first.

However, the Pilates matwork is designed to accommodate any level of fitness. Understanding that the Pilates method is a corrective system of exercise in which you will progress in stages is also key.

You must begin slowly, reading about and visualizing the movements. As you will not have the added benefit of a trainer to correct your form, it is important that you become aware of your body before beginning and throughout your progress. Do not push your body past the point of comfortable movement. These exercises are meant to teach you a new way to *connect* to your body, not to conquer it. Therefore, begin with only a few of the movements; the seven modified beginner exercises are meant to teach you the fundamentals that will apply not only to the rest of the program but also to the way you move in general. Learn them well and you will progress in no time.

What kind of a mat should I use and where?

Any mat or pad that is thick or dense enough to support and protect the delicate vertebrae of your spine will do. A thick carpet or long, folded blanket may also do the trick. As some of the exercises involve rolling back or pressing your spine into the mat, you will want to make sure you are not going to work out on a surface hard enough to bruise or injure your vertebrae. A surface that is too soft is not desirable, either, because it inhibits balance.

The beauty of the Pilates matwork is that it can be done anywhere your body can fit at full length. You need no special accoutrements or equipment to master the principles of this well-designed method.

What should I wear?

Workout clothing (leggings, tank tops, and so on) is the most practical and will allow you to see the muscles you are working, but any comfortable clothing will do. No shoes or sneakers are necessary. Don't wear pants with belt loops or anything that may irritate your back while performing the movements of the matwork.

When is the best time to do the matwork?

Doing the exercises is what's important; it matters less when you do them.

Some people prefer to begin their day with the matwork to wake up, and some use it to relieve stress at the end of their day. Some like it before lunch. And some will do little bits throughout their day. The bottom line is to make sure that you are doing at least some of the movements every day. Try to integrate the principles of the method into your daily schedule and you will find that you increase your strength, awareness, and flexibility faster than you thought imaginable.

It is not recommended that you exercise directly after eating, when you are sick, or if you are overtired. As the movements rely upon the utmost concentration in order to be truly effective, it is important to be clearheaded when doing the exercises. Remember that one well-performed movement is more effective and less destructive than twenty sloppy ones.

How many times a week should I do the matwork and for how long?

Joseph Pilates used to recommend committing to the matwork four times a week for fifteen to thirty minutes at a go. This number will change in stages. Some longtime students of the mat can perform the entire advanced sequence in fifteen minutes and not sacrifice the precision of the movements. The most important element of working with the Pilates method is precision and control; therefore, you must use your common sense to determine your own exercise time frame. In the beginning you may prefer to practice for half an hour. You may be strapped for time and do only five minutes. In either case you must be sure to limit the quantity of exercises to match the quality with which you perform them.

HOW TO USE THIS BOOK

The Pilates Body is laid out in stages so that you can achieve the most possible from an at-home program.

Begin with the basic modified mat (see "Getting Started") and practice until you feel confident in your body's ability to take the next step. From there you can begin building your way up in the full program. Do not try to add too many new exercises at once. Remember, it is the quality with which you perform each exercise that counts!

Remember to read all the instructions thoroughly before beginning. Visualize the movements as you read the descriptions, and then use the photos and visual cues as your reference thereafter. There are always things that get missed the first time around, so periodically come back to the instructions as you progress, and reevaluate your form and knowledge. Have a friend help by checking your positions against the instructions in the book. Or try teaching some of the basic exercises to a friend. Both of these are good ways to stay on top of the learning process. Lastly, try to find a certified Pilates instructor to work with in your area. (A list of certified instructors and studios is provided on p.174.)

Along with step-by-step instructions I have included what I call the "Inside Scoop." The Inside Scoop is essentially a list of tips that I have derived from training hundreds of diverse clients. These tips are meant to aid in the efficiency of understanding the movement as well as being a checkpoint to help you avoid common bad habits. The Inside Scoop is the next best thing to having a trainer on hand, so use its information to become your own personal trainer.

The level of each exercise is clearly indicated, both in the text and in the use of different models.

- Follow Caitlin for all beginner exercises.

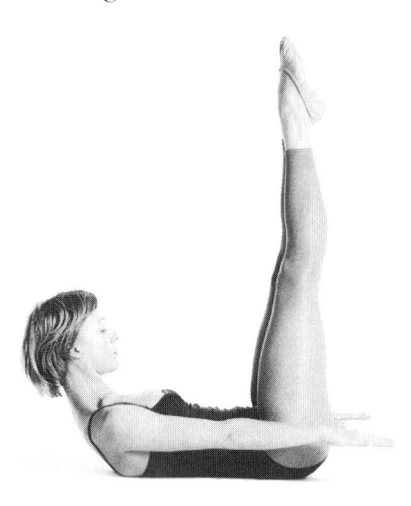

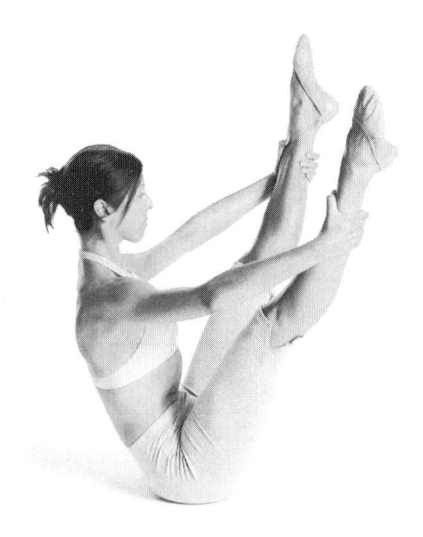

- Begin adding exercises with Dana as you progress to the intermediate level.

- And follow Julianna as you progress to the advanced exercises.

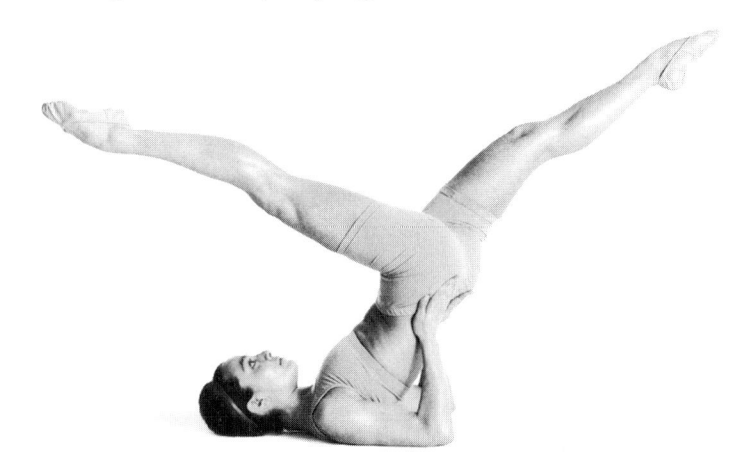

Add one new exercise at a time. Do not rush your progress.

As an added benefit, in each step-by-step description I have included instructions for transitioning from one exercise to the next to create the sequential element that makes the matwork fluid and rhythmic.

Remember that variations and tips on progressing are included throughout the text, so be sure to go back and read over the instructions when you feel ready to move on.

Please note: The models used in this book have been training in the Pilates method for years. Although their bodies may seem to represent an unrealistic ideal for many, they have worked hard to achieve their fitness goals. Above all else, they were chosen for their skill in exemplifying the movements during the long and arduous days of shooting. I hope in earnest that they do not intimidate but inspire.

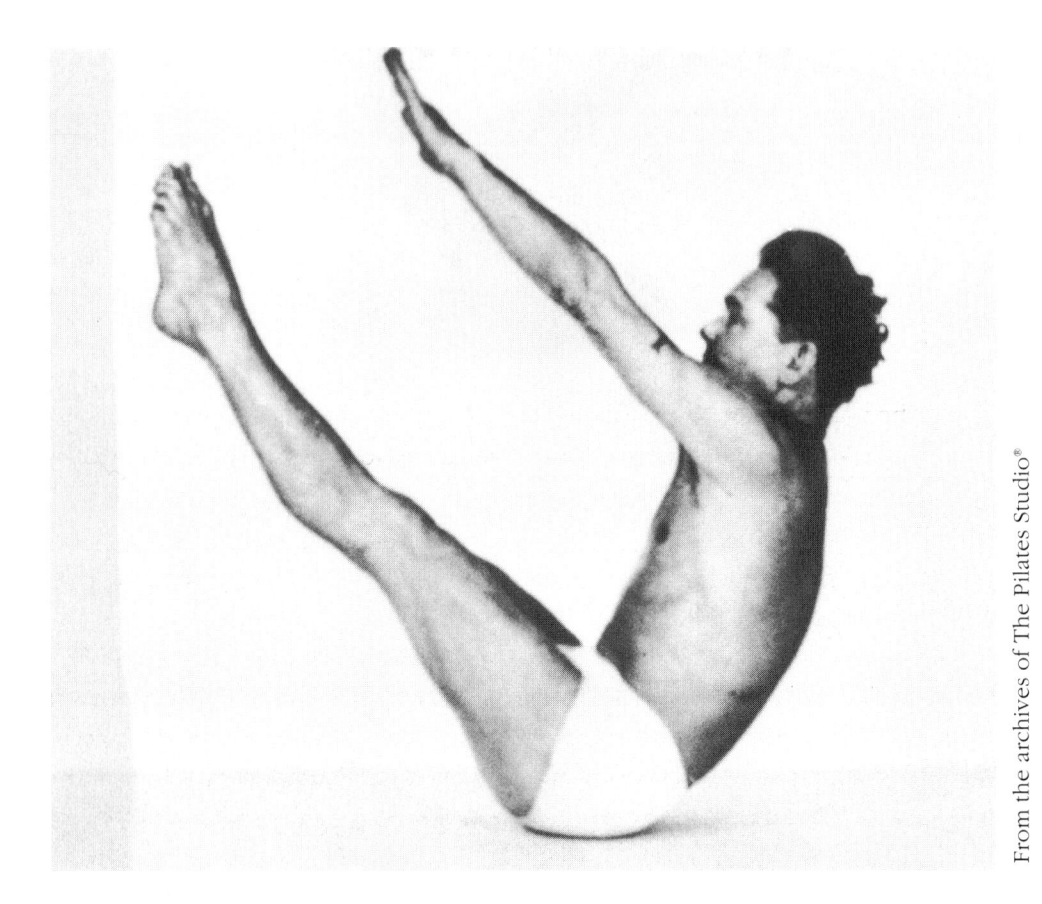

Joseph Pilates demonstrates the "Teaser."

From the archives of The Pilates Studio®

The Matwork

- *Getting Started—Modified Beginner Matwork:* These seven exercises should be your introduction to the mat for the first few weeks, or however long you still feel you are working within your range. Just because they are called beginner exercises does not mean they are easy, so don't be so eager to get on to the advanced stuff. Mastering the beginner matwork is the most challenging part of the program, and once you have done this, you will then be ready to add new exercises.
- *The Pilates Mat—Full Program:* All the exercises, beginner through advanced, are charted with step-by-step instructions, tips for performing the exercises, photos of the exercise movements, and creative visuals illustrating the key focal points of each exercise. Remember to listen to your body when adding a new movement. Nothing should ever hurt when performing the exercises. Take your time, use concentration and control, and enjoy the movements.
- *Advanced Extras:* These six exercises are adapted from the exercises most commonly performed on the apparatus. They are for the advanced student who wishes to add new movements to his/her program. They should be performed with the same caution and control as the rest of the matwork. Just because you are advanced does not mean you are above injuring yourself. Remember to work from your powerhouse and listen to your body.
- *The Standing Arm Series:* This series need not be performed in its entirety. Choose from the variety of exercises in this section to create a balanced addition to your mat workout.
- *The Wall (Cooldown):* The Wall is meant as the cooldown section of the program. Its movements, especially Rolling Down the Wall, can be used throughout the day to stretch and relax the muscles of your back, neck, and shoulders.

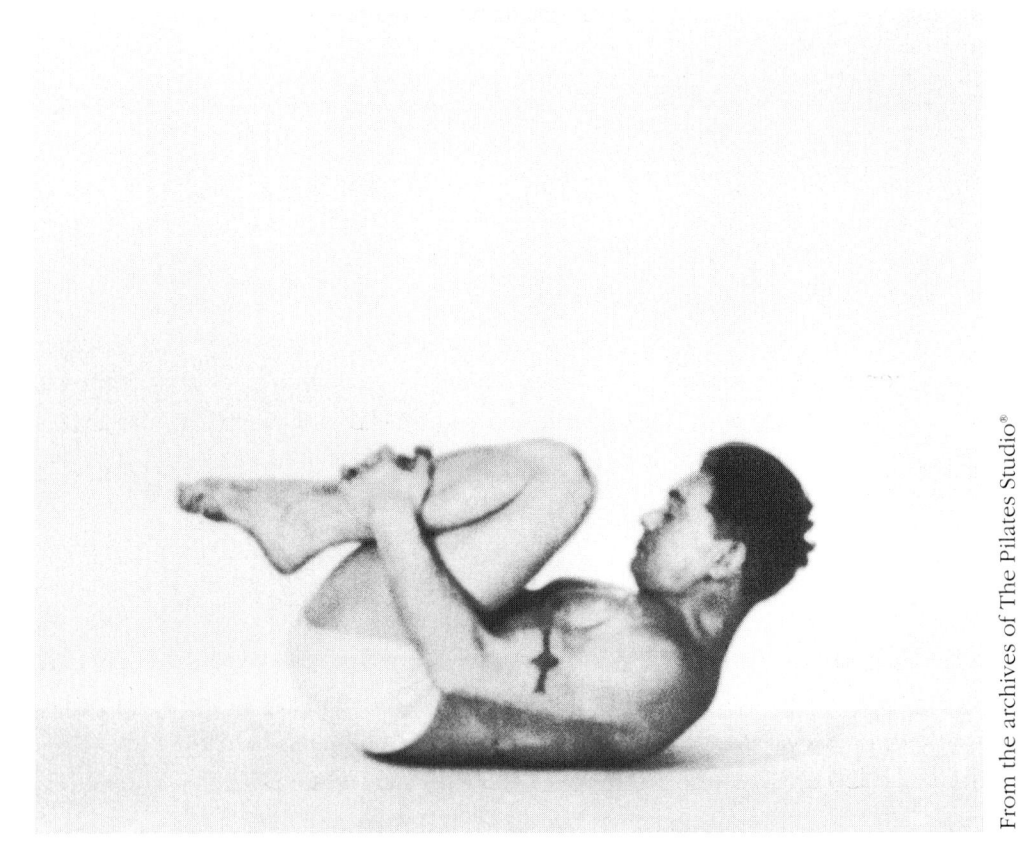

Joseph Pilates demonstrates the "Double Leg Stretch."

Getting Started:
Modified Beginner Matwork

The goal of the modified beginning section is to introduce your body to the movements of the matwork in a safe and effective way. The focus of these seven exercises is on finding the muscles of your powerhouse—abdominals, buttocks, lower back, and hips—and strengthening them to support you through the more complicated movements to come.

Make sure to stay attentive to what you are feeling as you introduce your body to the movements and as you discover new muscles. The modified beginning seven will be the foundation upon which your knowledge, understanding, and power builds, so make your best effort to stay consistent and aware.

Remember to come back to the beginning seven every so often to redefine your progress and get back to the core of the technique. These seven exercises are also great to use when you travel and need a quick fitness fix.

MODIFIED BEGINNER

THE HUNDRED

Step by Step

1. Lie on your back with your knees bent in toward your chest. Deeply inhale, and as you exhale feel your chest and belly sinking into the mat beneath you.
2. Keep that *feeling of a weight pressing your torso down into the mat* as you bring your head up to look at your belly button. (Make sure you are folding forward from your upper torso and not your neck.)
3. Lift forward until you feel the bottom of your shoulder blades pressing into the mat beneath you.
4. Stretch your arms out beside you, reaching from deep in the pit of your arm, *as if you were trying to touch the wall across the room with your fingertips.*
5. Begin pumping your arms straight up and down *as if you were slapping water.* (Keep your arms straight and pumping just above the mat.)
6. Inhale for five counts and exhale for five counts, reaching ever forward as you breathe.
7. Maintain this position, pumping your arms and breathing, for as close to one hundred counts as you can manage.
8. End by lowering your head and placing the soles of your feet flat on the mat to prepare for the Roll-Up. . . .

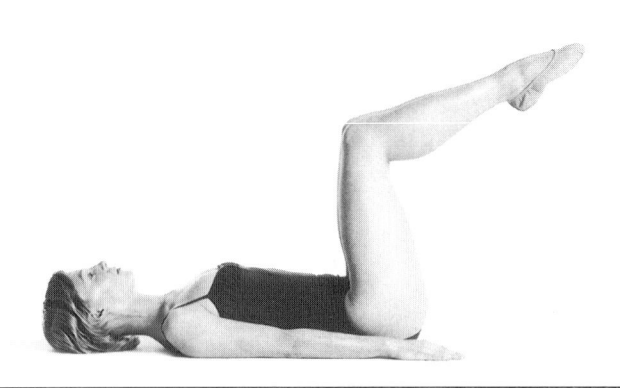

The Hundred is a breathing exercise. It is meant to begin circulating your blood to warm up the body in preparation for the exercises to follow.

The Beginning Scoop

GOAL
- To stay lifted in your head and chest region for all one hundred breaths. You should be able to maintain a flat back and "scooped" belly throughout.

FOCUS
- Make sure you are always focused on the weight of your belly as it sinks into your spine.
- Keep your shoulders pressing away from your ears to stretch the neck muscles and increase the abdominal focus.
- Squeezing the buttocks and knees together will provide stability for your lower back.

NO-NOS
- If your neck hurts, put it down. Do not push to the point of strain.
- Do not push your abdominals out or hold your breath as you go.
- Do not let your thighs rest on your chest as you perform the movements.

BEGINNING MODIFICATIONS
- You can place a small pillow or rolled towel under your head to support your neck if it is too difficult to hold lifted.
- Begin with twenty or thirty breaths and gradually increase to one hundred.

BEGINNING PROGRESSIONS
- As you progress, allow the exhalations to get longer and longer in order to improve your cardiovascular capacity.
- Begin trying to straighten your legs to the ceiling at a ninety-degree angle as you continue pumping your arms.

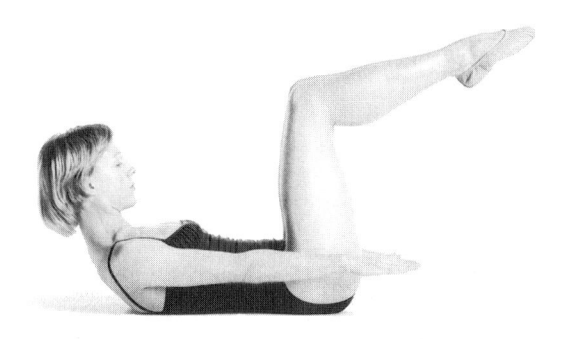

MODIFIED BEGINNER

THE ROLL-UP

Step by Step

1. Lie on your back with your knees together and bent and the soles of your feet planted firmly on the mat. Your arms are long by your sides.
2. Squeezing your knees together and tightening your buttocks, inhale and roll up by bringing your chin to your chest and continuing forward.
3. Exhale as you straighten your legs and stretch forward. Keep your navel pulling back into your spine. This is opposition at work!
4. In order to feel the articulation of your spine, it is helpful to imagine this rhythm: Lift your chin to your chest, lift your chest over your ribs, lift your ribs over your belly, lift your belly over your hips, and imagine trying to lift up out of your hips and over your thighs as you stretch forward.
5. Initiate rolling back down by squeezing your buttocks and slightly tucking your tailbone underneath you as you bend your knees. Pull your navel deeper into your spine.
6. Reverse the sequence of the exercise and exhale as you feel each vertebra pressing into the mat beneath you. Keep squeezing your knees together for stability.
7. When the backs of your shoulders touch the mat, lower your head and bring your arms down by your sides.
8. Repeat this sequence three to five times and finish by lying flat on the mat with your arms long by your sides to prepare for Single Leg Circles. . . .

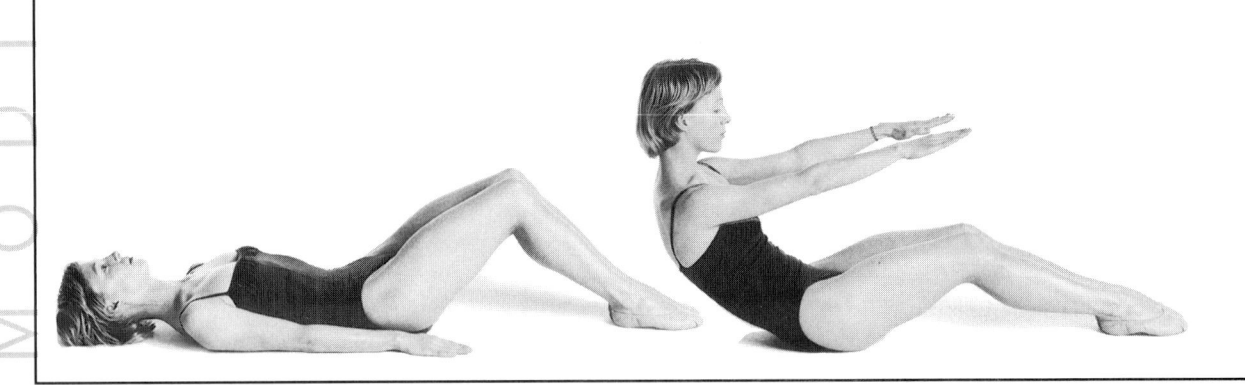

The Roll-Up works the powerhouse and stretches the hamstrings.

The Beginning Scoop

GOAL
- To engage the muscles of your powerhouse and flow through the movements.

FOCUS
- The key to this exercise is rhythm. Try to feel the fluidity of the sequence.
- Use your breath to help control your movements.
- Remember to squeeze your legs together to keep your lower body still.
- Keep your chin tucked into your chest as you roll up and back down so that you are not pulling from your neck. Think of curling yourself forward, stretching, and then *slowly* uncurling back down to the mat.
- Remember to use the oppositional force of pulling back in your belly as you stretch forward.

NO-NOS
- Do not allow your feet to lift off the mat as you roll up and lower yourself back down.
- Do not use your shoulders to pull you up.
- Do not allow your body to flop forward as you stretch.

BEGINNING MODIFICATIONS
- If you have trouble rolling up, pull yourself up by placing your hands on the underside of the legs. Remember to still squeeze the legs together for support and pull your navel into your spine. (Make sure your feet are not too close to your buttocks or you will not have the range of motion to be able to come up.)
- Squeeze a ball or small pillow between your ankles to help stabilize your lower body throughout.

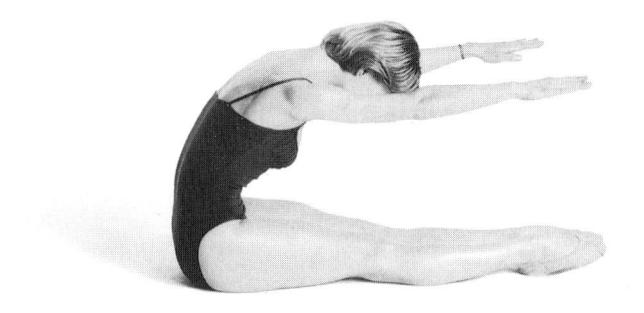

MODIFIED BEGINNER

SINGLE LEG CIRCLES

Step by Step

1. Lie on your back with your knees bent, the soles of your feet firmly planted, and your arms long by your sides. Feel your entire spine pressing into the mat beneath you.
2. Straighten one leg up to the ceiling at a ninety-degree angle and turn it out slightly in the hip socket. (This will help you to maintain contact between the back of your hip and the mat.)
3. Begin the circle by moving your leg *across your body first,* then circling it down, around, and back up to its starting position. Do not let your leg swing too far outside your hip joint.
4. *Imagine your leg is a heavy lead pole and you are scratching circles into the ceiling with it.*
5. The accent of this movement is on the "upswing." Press your navel deep into your spine to bring your leg back up, but do not lift your buttocks off the mat.
6. Complete three to five repetitions, inhaling as you begin the motion and exhaling as you complete it. Reverse the direction of the leg, making sure you remain stabilized in your hips at all times—that is, try not to let the hips wobble as you circle the leg.
7. Repeat the sequence with your other leg.
8. End by bending both knees, feet flat on the mat, and rolling up to a sitting position. Lift your bottom forward to your heels to prepare for Rolling Like a Ball. . . .

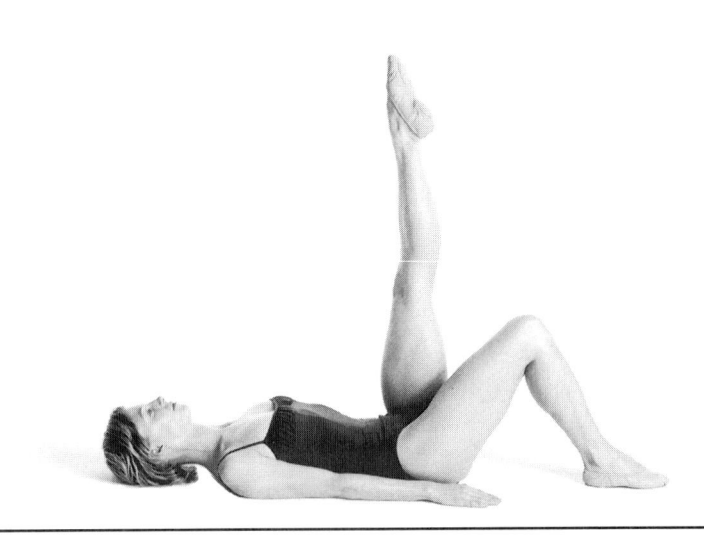

The Single Leg Circles articulate, stretch, and strengthen your leg in the hip joint.

The Beginning Scoop

- To remain perfectly still in your upper body and control the circling movement from your powerhouse.
- The accent for this exercise is on the upswing. Try to hold your leg steady at the end of each circle to feel your abdominals at work.
- Press your palms into the mat for added stability.
- You want to feel this exercise working the inner and outer thighs as well as the powerhouse region.
- In order to stop the quadriceps (thigh) muscle from doing all the work, turn your leg out slightly in the hip and think of engaging your buttock to help perform the movement.
- Make sure that you do not drop the leg so low as to cause your back to arch off the mat.
- Make sure that your knee does not turn inward as you circle the leg. Think of leading with the *inside* of your knee instead.
- As you progress, you can gradually increase the size of your circles. Make sure to maintain control in the hips throughout.

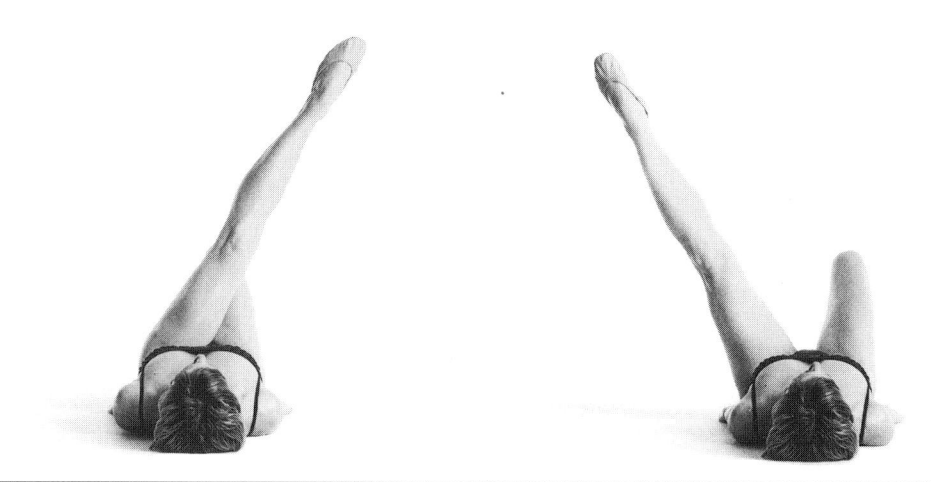

MODIFIED BEGINNER

ROLLING LIKE A BALL

Step by Step

1. Sit at the front of your mat with your knees bent toward your chest and open slightly.
2. Place a hand under each thigh (not behind your knees) and lift your feet off the mat until you are balancing on your tailbone. Your chin is tucked into your chest, your elbows are wide, and you should feel you have taken on the roundness of a ball.
3. Initiate the rolling by sinking your navel deep into your spine and falling backward, bringing your legs with you. Do not throw your head back to begin the momentum; work instead from deep within your abdominal muscles.
4. Inhale as you roll back and exhale as you come forward, placing emphasis on keeping a uniform distance between your chest and thighs as you go. Keep your elbows extended so that you work from your abdominals and not your shoulders.
5. *Imagine you are in a rocking chair that is about to tip over, and quickly bring yourself back to a balanced position.*
6. Repeat the Rolling Like a Ball five or six times and end by putting the soles of your feet flat on the mat and lifting your bottom back and away from your heels to prepare for the Single Leg Stretch. . . .

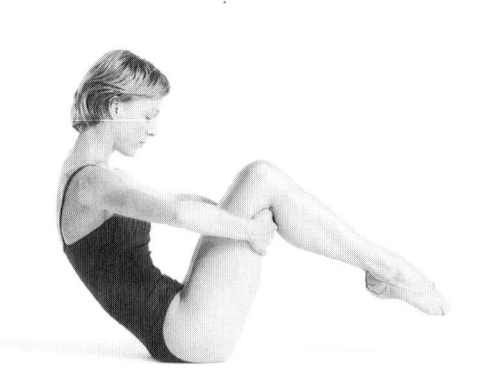

Rolling Like a Ball works on your abdominals, improves balance, and acts as a spinal massage.

The Beginning Scoop

- To stay completely rounded throughout the rolling movement.
- Momentum is the key here. The more slowly you roll back, the less chance you have of making it back up.
- Try to allow yourself to feel each vertebra as it presses back into the mat, like running up the scale on a xylophone.
- Remember to pull your abdominals in, and to keep your head and neck supported throughout the rolling movement.
- Each time you come forward, "put on the brakes" and balance on your tailbone. (Do not allow your feet to touch the mat.)

- Do not roll back onto your neck; think of stopping at the bottom of the shoulder blades instead.
- Make sure you do not allow your head to fly back and forth throughout the movement. Keep it securely tucked toward your knees.
- Do not close your eyes as it inhibits balance.

- Test your strength by placing a ball (about the size of a basketball) between your scooped belly and thighs and see if you can still perform the sequence.

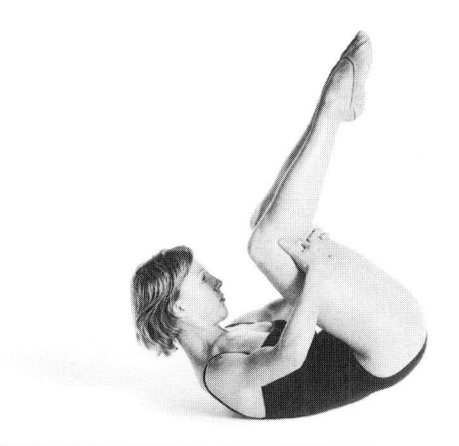

MODIFIED BEGINNER

SINGLE LEG STRETCH

Step by Step

1. Lie on your back with your knees pulled into your chest.
2. Grab hold of one shin with both hands and extend your other leg to the ceiling at as close to a ninety-degree angle as you can manage. If your right leg is bent, place your right hand on your ankle and your left hand on your knee.
3. With your elbows extended, lift your head and neck and reach your chin toward your belly.
4. Exhale and watch as your navel sinks deep into your spine. Hold it there *as if you were anchored to the mat below*.
5. Inhale and switch legs and hand positions. Stretch your extended leg long out of your hip and in line with the center of your body.
6. Repeat three sets of the Single Leg Stretch and then pull both knees into your chest to prepare for the Double Leg Stretch. . . .

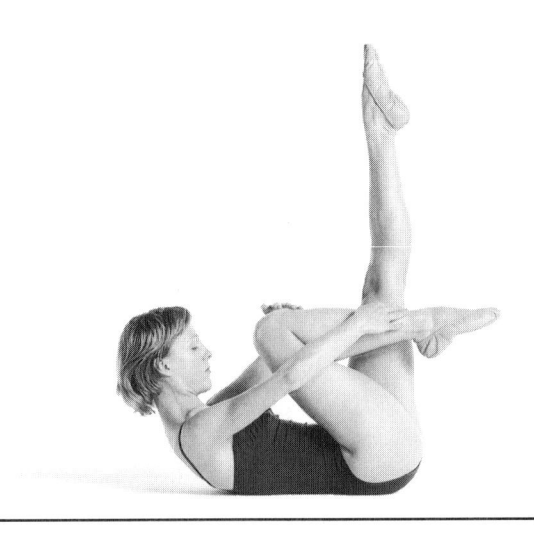

The Single Leg Stretch works your powerhouse and stretches your back and legs.

The Beginning Scoop

- To stay completely still in your upper body as you perform the movements of the legs.
- Remember to stay lifted from your abdominals and the back of your chest area. Scoop your belly at all times and press your spine *further* into the mat as you switch legs.
- Keep your elbows extended and your shoulders pressing down and away from your ears in order to best utilize your abdominals.
- Keep your extended leg at a height that enables you to maintain a flat back.
- Squeezing the buttocks as you extend your leg will help ensure the integrity of the position.
- Do not let your shoulders creep up around your ears.
- Do not lift your head from the neck itself. (If your neck gets tired, rest it back down on the mat and then try again to lift correctly.)
- Do not release your abdominal muscles as you switch legs.

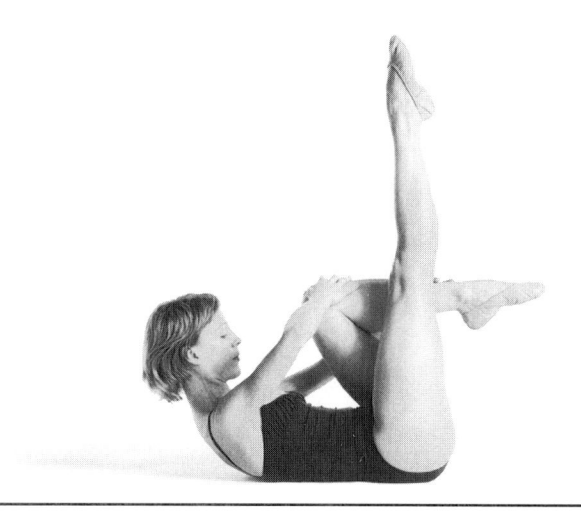

MODIFIED BEGINNER

DOUBLE LEG STRETCH

Step by Step

1. Lie on your back with both knees pulled into your chest.
2. Extend your elbows and bring your head and neck up with your chin reaching for your belly.
3. Exhale and watch as your navel sinks deep into your spine.
4. Inhale deeply and stretch your body long, reaching your arms back by your ears and your legs straight up to the ceiling at a ninety-degree angle *as if you were stretching before getting out of bed in the morning.*
5. *Imagine keeping your torso firmly anchored to the mat, as you did in the Single Leg Stretch, and do not allow your head to move from your chest.*
6. As you exhale, draw your knees back into your chest by circling your arms around to meet them.
7. Pull your knees deeply into your chest to increase the emphasis on the exhalation, as if you were squeezing the air out of your lungs.
8. Repeat the sequence five times, remaining still in your torso as you inhale to stretch and exhale to pull.
9. End by pulling both knees into your chest with a deep exhalation and then roll up to sitting to prepare for the Spine Stretch Forward. . . .

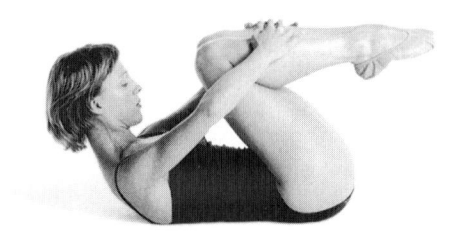

The Double Leg Stretch works the powerhouse and stretches the arms and legs.

The Beginning Scoop

- To remain perfectly still in your center, chin into chest, throughout the movements.
- Keep your neck supported by staying completely still in the upper body as you perform the movement. Squeeze your buttocks and inner thighs together tightly as you extend your legs to support your lower back.
- As you inhale and stretch out, make sure your arms are straight and you are reaching in opposition. (Feel as if you are being pulled in two directions with only your abdominals to hold you down on the mat.)
- If you pull your chest up to your knees very deeply as you exhale and keep your elbows extended, you will feel a nice release stretch in the trapezius region (upper back and neck area). This is generally a very tense spot on most people, so enjoy the release as you exhale.
- Do not let your head fall back as you stretch your arms above your head.

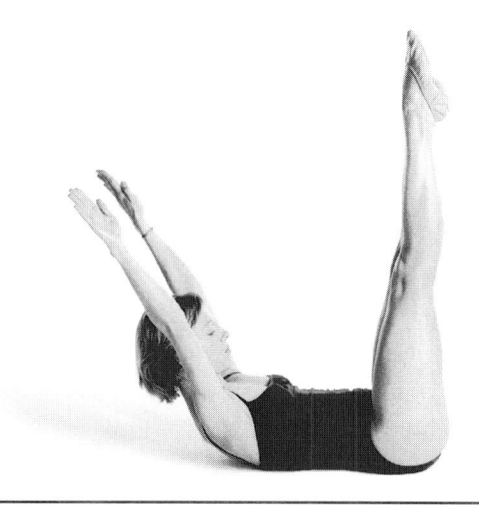

MODIFIED BEGINNER

SPINE STRETCH FORWARD

Step by Step

1. Sit up tall with your legs extended on the mat in front of you and open to slightly wider than your hips' width. Bend your knees slightly to release your hamstrings.
2. Straighten your arms out in front of you at shoulder height and flex your feet. Inhale and sit even taller.
3. Bring your chin to your chest and begin rolling down, pressing your navel deep into your spine as you round. *Imagine you are forming the letter C with your body.*
4. Exhale as you stretch your upper body forward, resisting the stretch by pulling back with your abdominals. This is opposition at work again. Your hips should remain still at all times.
5. Inhale as you reverse the motion of the exercise, *rolling up as if constrained by a wall behind you.*
6. Exhale, returning to your tall seated position. Press your shoulders down, and *stretch your back flat up against the imagined wall behind you.*
7. Repeat three times with the goal of increasing the stretch down the spine with each repetition.

Practice these seven modified exercises until you feel ready to move on to the basic exercises of the full mat program. . . .

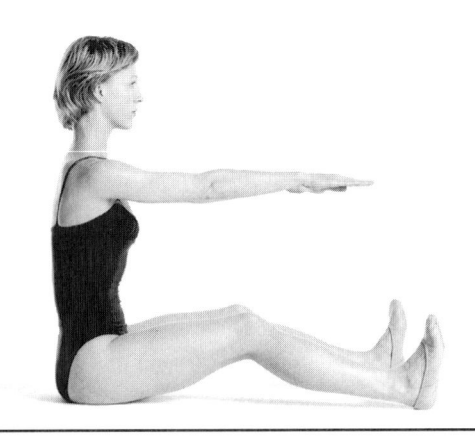

The Spine Stretch Forward works the deep abdominals, articulates the spine, and enhances good posture.

The Beginning Scoop

GOAL
- To keep your hips stable as you stretch your spine.

FOCUS
- Breathing is the key to a good stretch, so do not hold your breath, as this creates more tension in your body and limits your progress.
- Press your shoulders down and away from your ears as you roll yourself back up to release the muscles in the back of your neck. (The crown of your head should be stretching toward the ceiling.)
- As you stretch up to a tall seated position make sure you are initiating from your powerhouse and not lifting your head to come up. (Your head should be the last part up.)

NO-NOS
- Do not let your knees roll inward as you stretch forward. Think of pulling your baby toes back toward you as you stretch.
- Do not flop forward as you stretch. Think of reaching in opposition instead.
- Roll not back but up as you sit tall.

BEGINNING PROGRESSION
- As you progress, try to increase the stretch in your hamstrings by straightening one leg and then the other as you exhale forward.

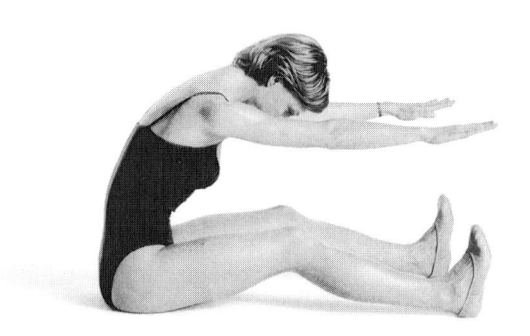

The Pilates Mat:
Full Program

THE EXERCISE SEQUENCE OF THE MAT

Remember that these exercises were developed as a sequence to create a flow of movement. Study this chart and try to visualize the transitions from one exercise to the next.

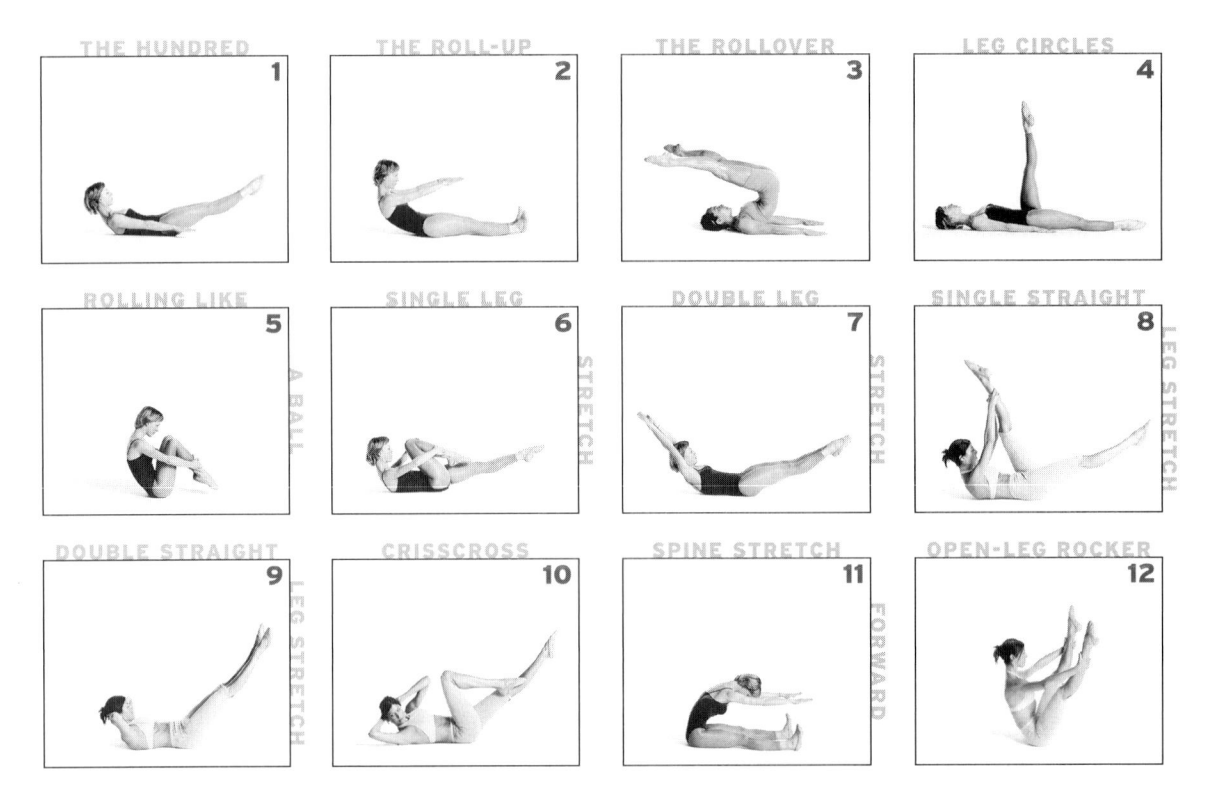

1. THE HUNDRED	2. THE ROLL-UP	3. THE ROLLOVER	4. LEG CIRCLES
5. ROLLING LIKE A BALL	6. SINGLE LEG STRETCH	7. DOUBLE LEG STRETCH	8. SINGLE STRAIGHT LEG STRETCH
9. DOUBLE STRAIGHT LEG STRETCH	10. CRISSCROSS	11. SPINE STRETCH FORWARD	12. OPEN-LEG ROCKER

50

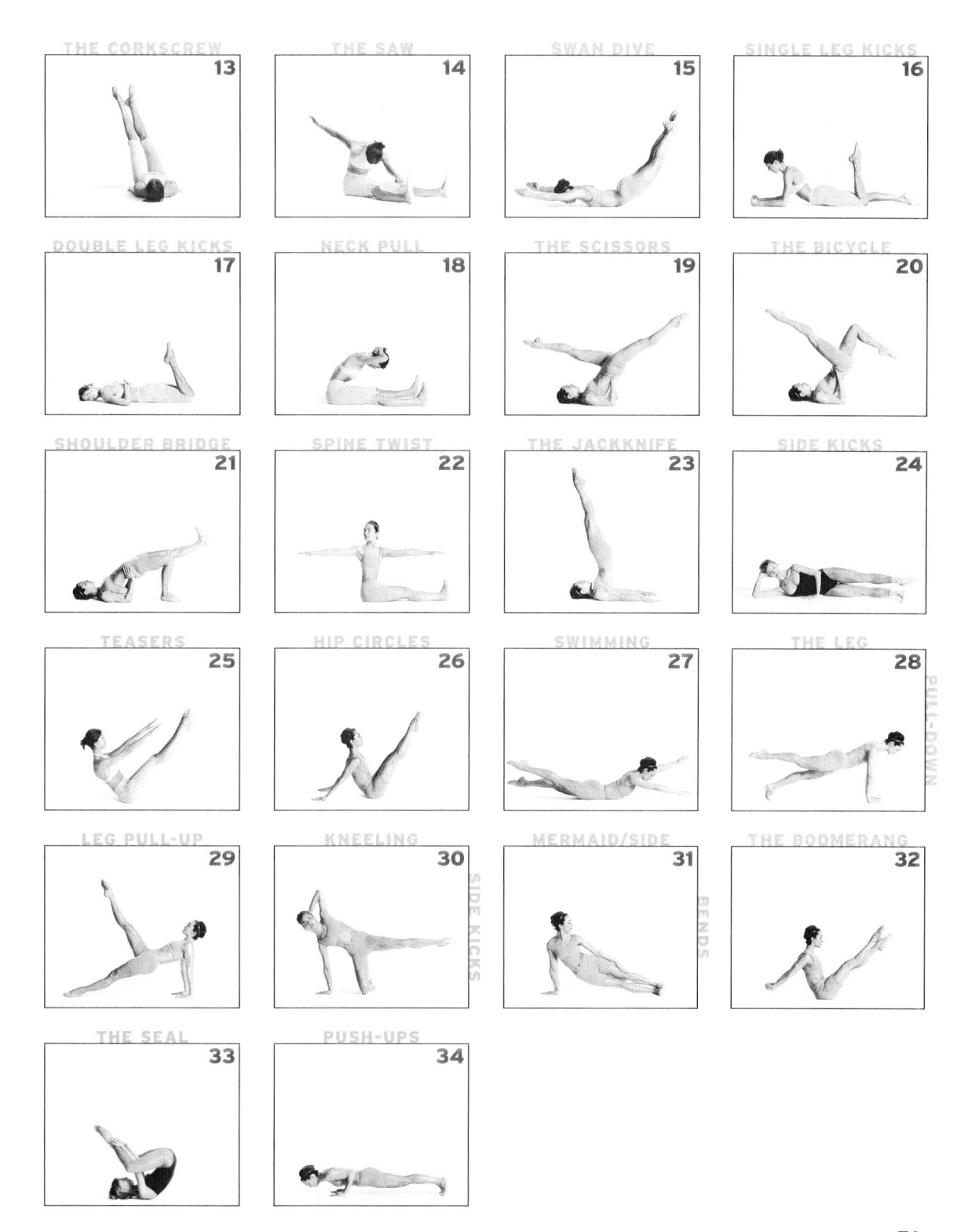

THE CORKSCREW **13**	THE SAW **14**	SWAN DIVE **15**	SINGLE LEG KICKS **16**
DOUBLE LEG KICKS **17**	NECK PULL **18**	THE SCISSORS **19**	THE BICYCLE **20**
SHOULDER BRIDGE **21**	SPINE TWIST **22**	THE JACKKNIFE **23**	SIDE KICKS **24**
TEASERS **25**	HIP CIRCLES **26**	SWIMMING **27**	THE LEG PULL-DOWN **28**
LEG PULL-UP **29**	KNEELING SIDE KICKS **30**	MERMAID/SIDE BENDS **31**	THE BOOMERANG **32**
THE SEAL **33**	PUSH-UPS **34**		

BEGINNER

THE HUNDRED

Step by Step

1. Lie on your back and pull your knees into your chest. Inhale deeply, and as you exhale sink your chest and belly into the mat beneath you.
2. Keep that *feeling of a weight pressing your torso down* as you bring your head up to look at your belly. (Make sure you are folding forward from your upper back and not your neck.)
3. Stretch your arms long by your sides and reach forward until you feel the bottom of your shoulder blades sinking into the mat beneath you.
4. Straighten your legs to the ceiling, squeezing the buttocks and backs of the upper inner thighs together until no light comes through them.
5. *Begin pumping your arms straight up and down as if you were slapping water.* (Keep the movement slightly above the mat and your arms straight.)
6. Inhale for five counts and exhale for five counts, reaching ever forward as you breathe.
7. Lower your legs to a forty-five-degree angle, or to the point just before your spine arches off the mat.
8. Maintain this position, pumping your arms and breathing for one hundred counts.
9. End by lowering your head and bringing your knees back into your chest before stretching yourself out to full length to prepare for the Roll-Up. . . .

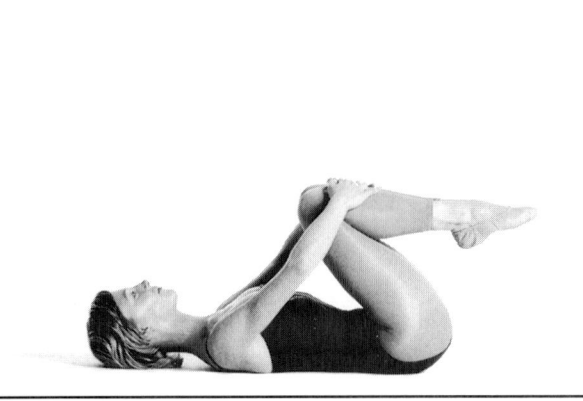

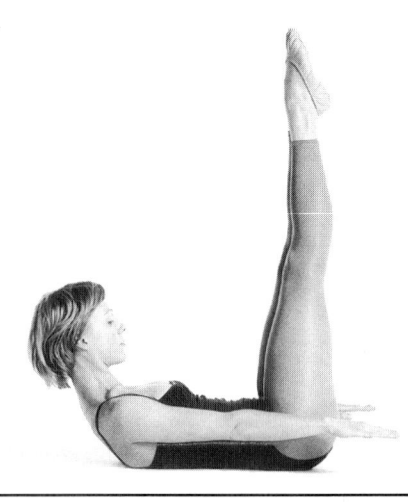

The Hundred is a breathing exercise meant to circulate your blood to warm up the body in preparation for the exercises to follow.

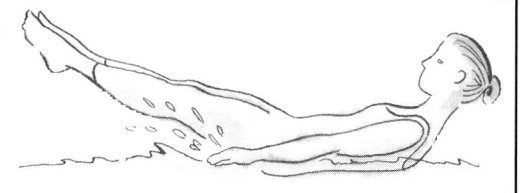

The Inside Scoop

- The goal of the Hundred is to be able to maintain a steady, flat back with your feet held at eye level. This is no easy task in the beginning, so do not push yourself to the point of strain.
- Make sure you are always focused on the weight of your belly as it sinks into your spine.
- Keep your shoulders pressing away from your ears to stretch the neck muscles and increase the abdominal focus.
- Squeezing the buttocks and backs of the upper inner thighs will provide stability for your lower back.
- Never drop your legs past the point of comfort for your back. You should be able to maintain a flat back and scooped belly throughout.
- If your lower back begins to hurt, simply bend your knees in toward your chest.
- If your neck hurts, rest it back down on the mat and then try again, making sure you are lifting from the area around the back of your chest and not from the neck itself.
- As you progress, allow your exhalations to get longer and longer in order to improve your cardiovascular capacity.

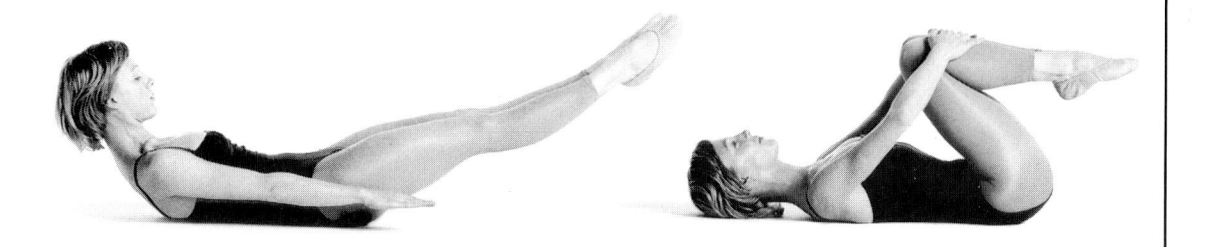

BEGINNER

THE ROLL-UP

Step by Step

1. Stretch out to your body's full length, *the way you might stretch your waking body as you get up in the morning.*
2. Squeeze your buttocks tightly and press the backs of your upper inner thighs together.
3. Flex your feet into the Pilates stance and bring your straight arms forward over your head.
4. As your arms pass over your chest, lift your head and inhale as you begin to roll up and forward.
5. *Imagine that your lower body is strapped down to the mat, stabilizing you just below the hip bones.*
6. In order to feel the articulation of your spine it is helpful to imagine this rhythm: Lift your chin to your chest, lift your chest up over your ribs, lift your ribs up over your belly, lift your belly up over your hips, and try to lift up out of your hips and over your thighs.
7. Exhale as you stretch forward from your hips while keeping your navel pulled back into your spine. This is opposition at work!
8. Initiate rolling back down by squeezing your buttocks and slightly tucking your tailbone underneath you. Inhale as you begin pulling your navel to your spine.
9. Reversing the sequence of the exercise, exhale as you feel each vertebra pressing into the mat beneath you. Keep squeezing the backs of your upper inner thighs together for stability.
10. When the backs of your shoulders touch the mat, lower your head and bring your arms over into a full-body stretch before beginning the movement again.
11. Complete three to five repetitions and end by lying flat on the mat with your arms long by your sides for the Rollover. . . .

    NOTE: If you are a beginner, go on to the Single Leg Circles. . . .

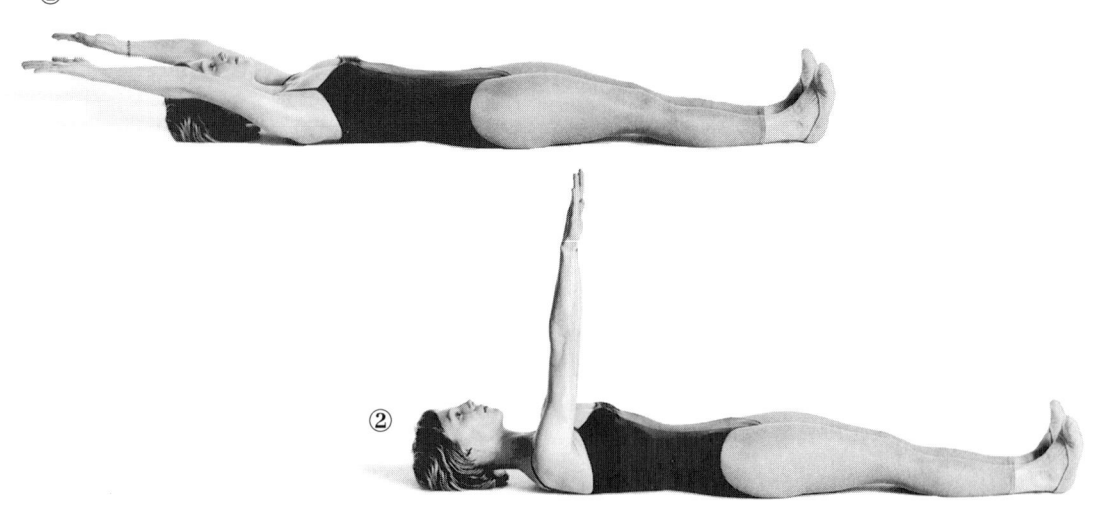

The Roll-Up stretches and strengthens the spine by articulating the vertebrae.

The Inside Scoop

GOAL
- To remain perfectly still in your lower body as you articulate your spine.

KEYS
- Try to feel the fluidity of the movement as you go.
- Use the oppositional forces of pulling back in your belly as you stretch forward so you do not flop.
- Remember to squeeze the backs of your upper inner thighs together to keep the lower body still. *Imagine you are gripping a small ball tightly between your ankles or the backs of your inner thighs.*
- Keep your chin tucked into your chest as you roll forward and back so that you are not pulling from your neck. Think of curling yourself forward, stretching, and then slowly uncurling back onto the mat, lengthening your spine as you go.

NO-NOS
- Do not roll up using your neck and shoulders. Use the muscles of your powerhouse.
- Do not allow your body to flop forward as you stretch.
- Do not allow your legs to lift off the mat as you roll up.

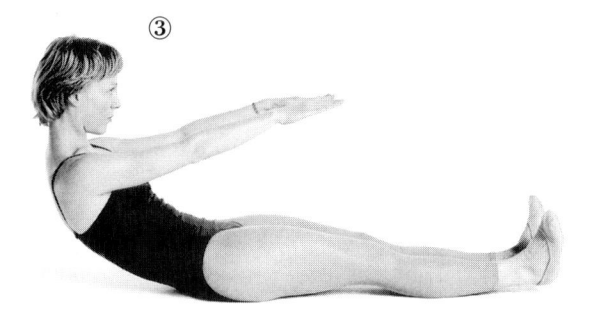

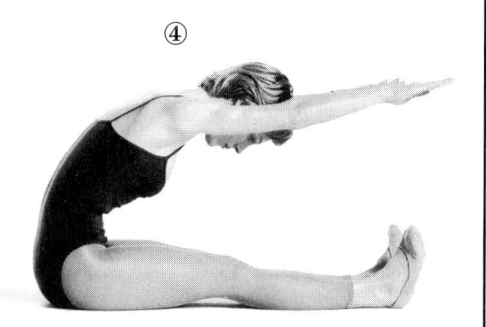

③

④

ADVANCED
THE ROLLOVER

Step by Step

1. Lie on the mat and extend your arms long by your sides for stability.
2. Initiate the Rollover by squeezing the buttocks and inhaling as you lift your legs off the mat and up over your head. Remember to lift from the back of your hips and control the movement with your powerhouse.
3. Roll over until your legs are parallel with the ceiling and mat. Do not roll onto the back of your neck. Balance on the back of the shoulders instead.
4. Open your legs to hip width and exhale as you roll your spine back down onto the mat, feeling each vertebra pressing into the mat as you go.
5. Control this movement by *imagining that your arms are lead bars pinning you to the mat*. Press weight into your palms to provide a frame in which you can align your body.
6. As you roll down, feel your spine stretching longer and longer by keeping your legs straight and slightly turned out.
7. When your tailbone has touched down, continue lowering the legs to the point just before your lower back arches off the mat. Squeeze your legs together again and repeat the Rollover sequence.
8. Complete three to five repetitions with the legs closed on the way over and open on the way down, and then reverse the leg position, completing three to five repetitions with the legs open on the way over and squeezing together on the way down.
9. Finish the Rollover by lying down with your arms long by your sides for the Single Leg Circles. . . .

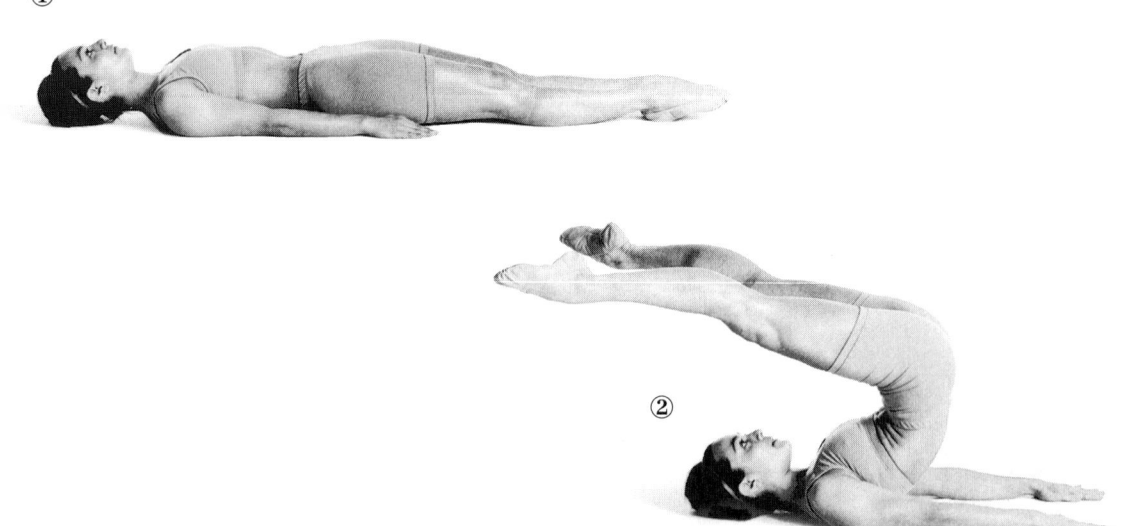

The Rollover stretches and articulates the spine by use of the powerhouse.

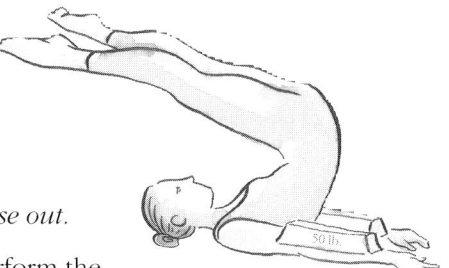

The Inside Scoop

If you have a bad neck or lower back, leave this exercise out.

- To keep your upper body glued to the mat as you perform the Rollover movements.

- Make sure you are suitably warmed up for this exercise.
- Fluidity! Use your powerhouse to keep the momentum steady throughout.
- Make sure you are lifting from the back of your hips and not simply allowing the weight of your legs to pull you over.
- Stabilize your torso by pressing weight into your palms and sliding them forward as you go.
- Keep a slight turnout at the hip and thigh to further increase your control.

- Never roll onto the back of your neck.
- If you cannot roll over without dropping your feet to the floor or bending your knees, you should not be doing this exercise yet.

- In the beginning you may "soften" your knees if the stretch in the back of your legs proves to be too much. (But don't make a habit of this!)

- For an additional stretch, place your toes on the mat overhead and press back into your heels.
- On the last Rollover you can bring your hands around overhead and grab your feet.

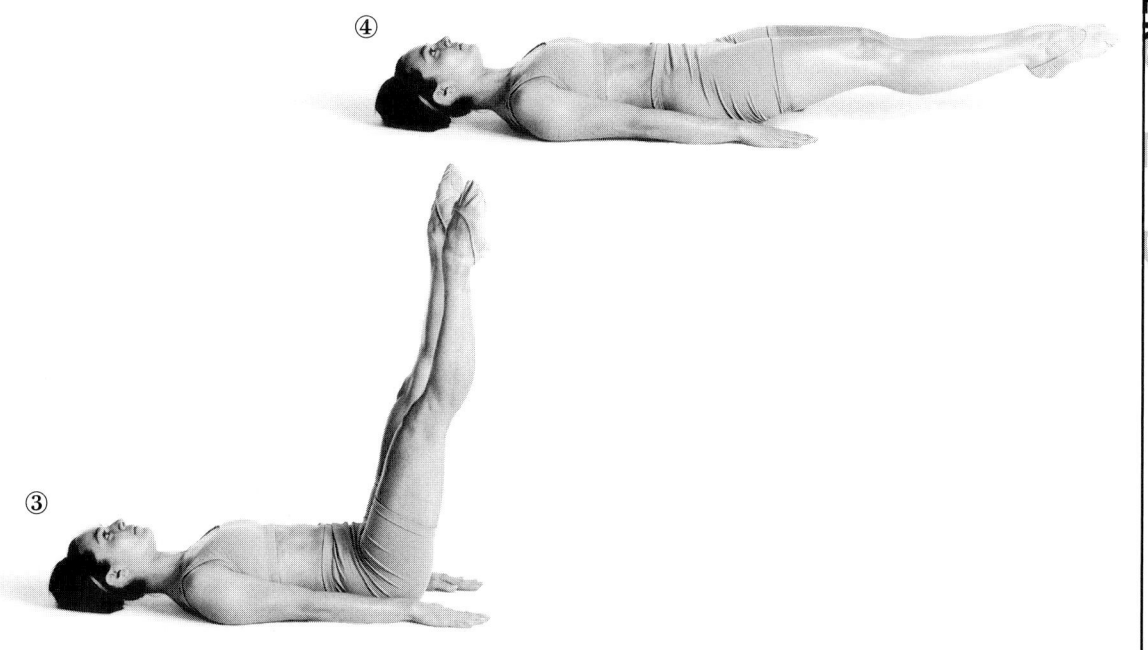

BEGINNER
SINGLE LEG CIRCLES

Step by Step

1. It helps to begin this exercise with a stretch by pulling one knee into your chest, then straightening it to the ceiling while holding your ankle or calf.
2. Bring your arms back down by your sides and leave your leg reaching straight up to the ceiling at as close to a ninety-degree angle as you can manage. Lengthen the back of your neck by pressing it to the mat.
3. Your opposite leg should be centered and reaching long in front of you for stability.
4. Stretch your leg across your body, then circle it down, around, and back up to its starting position. Keep your leg slightly turned out at your hip so that the back of your hip maintains contact with the mat. Do not allow your leg to swing too far to the outside of the hip joint.
5. *Imagine drawing circles on the ceiling with your leg.*
6. Complete three to five repetitions inhaling as you begin the motion and exhaling as you complete it. Then reverse the direction of your leg and complete three to five repetitions, making sure you remain stabilized in your hips at all times.
7. Repeat the stretch and circles with the other leg.
8. End the Single Leg Circles by bending both knees and rolling up to a sitting position. Lift your bottom forward to your heels to prepare for Rolling Like a Ball. . . .

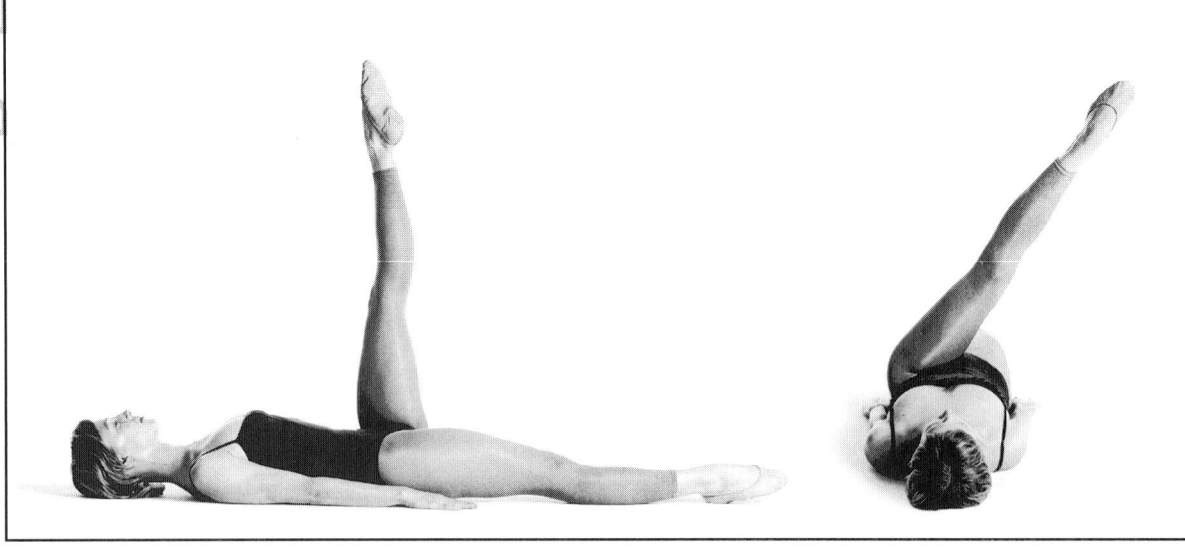

The Single Leg Circles articulate and strengthen the leg in the hip joint, and stretch the iliotibial band (muscle running along the outer part of the thigh).

The Inside Scoop

GOAL
- To remain completely still in your hips and torso as you circle your leg.

KEYS
- The accent for this exercise is on the upswing, where you must utilize your powerhouse to control the movement. Try to hold your leg steady at the end of each circle to feel your abdominals at work.
- Press your palms into the mat for added stability.
- In order to stop the quadriceps from doing all the work, turn your leg out slightly in the hip and think of engaging your buttock to help perform the movement. (If your hip clicks or pops, readjust your leg position and remember to squeeze your buttocks.)

NO-NOS
- Make sure that your knee does not turn inward as you circle the leg. Think of leading with the *inside* of your knee instead.
- Make sure that you do not drop your leg so low as to cause your back to arch off the mat. (If necessary, bend your opposite knee slightly to maintain a flat back.)
- Do not tilt your head back or lift the back of your chest off the mat.

PROGRESSION
- As you progress, you can gradually increase the size of your circles. Make sure to maintain control in the hips throughout!

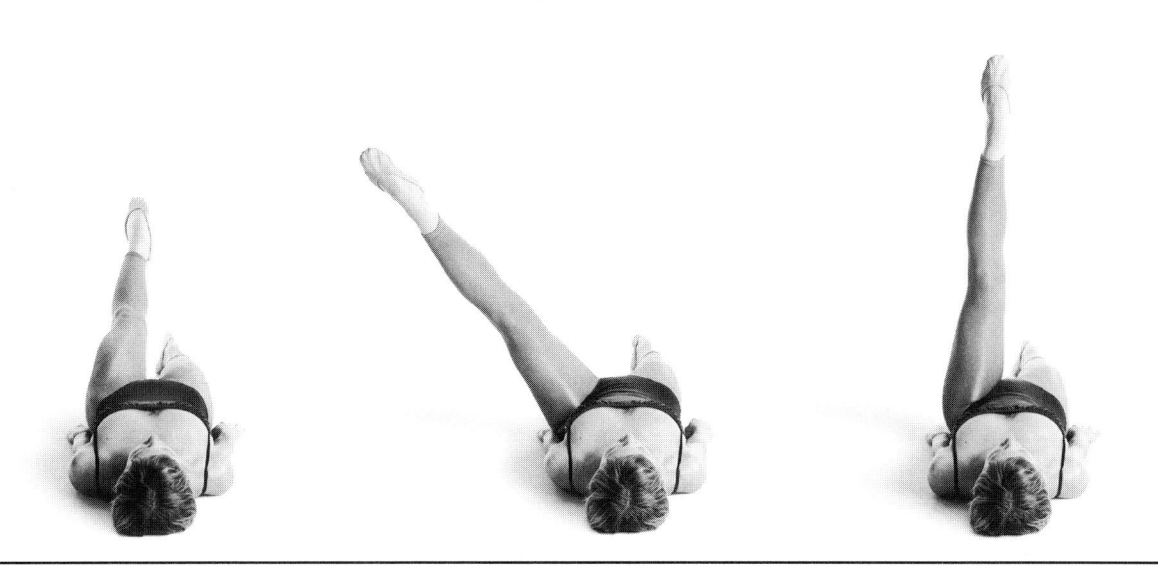

BEGINNER

ROLLING LIKE A BALL

Step by Step

1. Sit toward the front of your mat with your knees bent into your chest and grab your ankles. Keep your heels glued together and your elbows extended.
2. Open your knees slightly and lift your feet off the mat until you are balancing on your tailbone. Your chin is tucked into your chest and you should feel *you have taken on the roundness of a ball.*
3. Initiate the rolling by sinking your navel deep into your spine and falling backward, bringing your knees with you. Do not throw your head back to begin the movement.
4. Inhale as you roll back and exhale as you come forward, placing emphasis on pulling your heels in tightly to your buttocks as you come up.
5. *Imagine you are in a rocking chair that is about to tip over, and quickly bring yourself back up.*
6. Each time you come forward, "put on the brakes" and balance on your tailbone. Do not allow your feet to touch the mat.
7. Repeat the Rolling Like a Ball five or six times and prepare for the Stomach Series by sitting back on your mat and pulling one knee into your chest. . . .

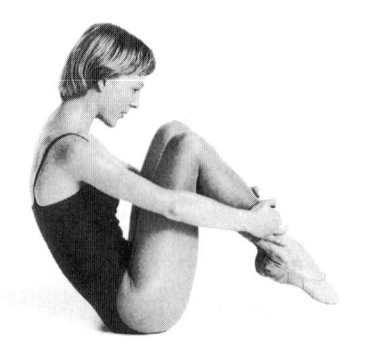

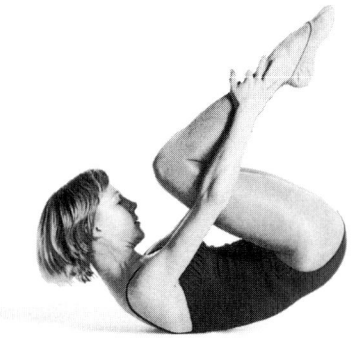

Rolling Like a Ball is an abdominal exercise that improves balance and massages the spine.

The Inside Scoop

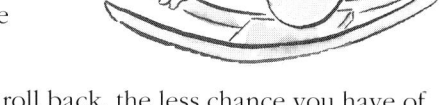

GOAL

- To stay as tightly tucked as possible throughout the entire movement.

KEYS

- Momentum is the key here. (The more slowly you roll back, the less chance you have of making it back up!)
- Try to feel each vertebra as it presses back into the mat, *like running up the scale of a xylophone.*
- Remember to pull your abdominals in and keep your head and neck supported throughout the rolling movement.
- Keep your elbows extended.

NO-NOS

- Do not allow your head to fly back and forth throughout the movement. Keep it securely tucked into your knees.
- Do not roll back onto your neck; think of stopping at the bottom of the shoulder blades instead.
- Do not allow your shoulders to creep up around your ears.

PROGRESSION

- For an added challenge, try placing your head between your knees and wrapping your arms around your legs instead of holding at the ankles.

As you progress be sure that your heels stay glued to your bottom throughout the rolling movement.

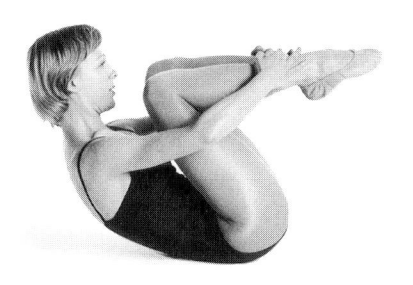

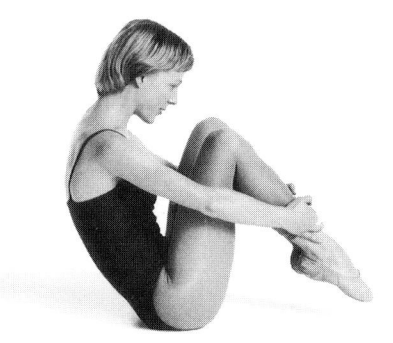

BEGINNER

SINGLE LEG STRETCH

Step by Step

1. Sit in the center of your mat with your knees bent. Take hold of your right leg and pull it into your chest with your inside hand on the knee and your outside hand on the ankle. (This will keep your leg in proper alignment with your hip.)
2. Roll your back down to the mat, bringing your bent leg with you.
3. Extend your opposite leg out in front of you and hold it above the mat at an angle that allows your back to remain flat on the mat.
4. With your elbows extended and your chin lifted onto your chest, inhale and watch as your navel sinks deep into your spine.
5. *Imagine you are anchored into the floor below.*
6. Exhale and switch legs, bringing the outside hand to the ankle and the inside hand to the knee. Stretch your extended leg long out of your hip and in line with the center of your body.
7. Repeat five to ten sets of the Single Leg Stretch and then pull both knees into your chest and go on to the Double Leg Stretch. . . .

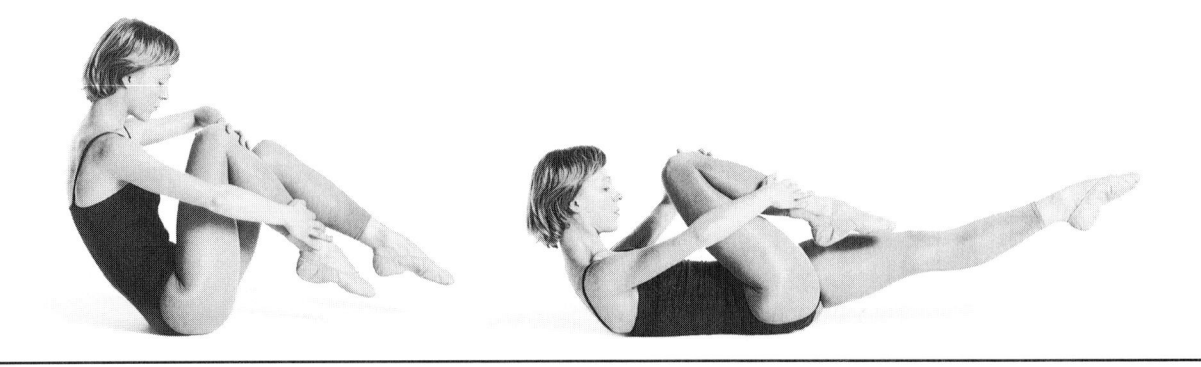

This is the first of five exercises termed the "Stomach Series." They are meant to flow from one to the next without changing the initial body position.

The Inside Scoop

GOAL
- To stay lifted and perfectly still in your torso as you perform the sequence.

KEYS
- Stay lifting forward from the abdominals and the back of your chest. (Keep your eyes on your belly.)
- Scoop your belly in at all times and press your spine *further* into the mat as you switch legs.
- Keep your elbows extended and your shoulders pressing down and away from your ears in order to best utilize your abdominals.
- Squeezing the buttocks as you extend your leg will help ensure the integrity of your leg position.

NO-NOS
- Do not lift forward from the neck itself.
- Make sure you are not lowering your extended leg below hip level. Keep it at a height that enables you to maintain a flat back.

MODIFICATIONS
- If you have a bad knee, hold the underside of the thigh instead of the top of the knee.
- For a bad back, extend the straight leg to the ceiling only. As your lower abdominal strength improves, you will be able to begin lowering it to a more challenging angle.

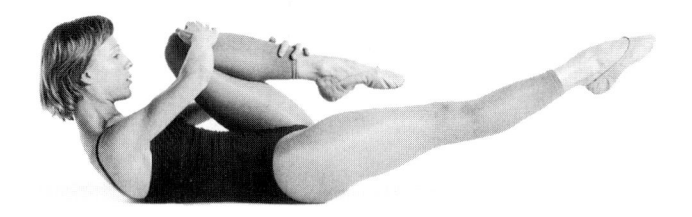

BEGINNER — SINGLE LEG STRETCHER

BEGINNER

DOUBLE LEG STRETCH

Step by Step

1. Lie on your back and pull both knees into your chest, elbows extended and head lifted.
2. Inhale deeply and stretch your body long, reaching your arms back by your ears and with your legs long out in front of you and raised off the mat at about a forty-five-degree angle, *as if you were stretching before getting out of bed in the morning.*
3. *Imagine your torso firmly anchored to the mat,* as you did in the Single Leg Stretch, and do not allow your head to move off your chest.
4. As you exhale, draw your knees back into your chest by circling your arms around to meet them.
5. Sink your belly further from your knees to increase the emphasis on the exhalation, as if you were compressing air out of your lungs.
6. Repeat the sequence five to ten times, remaining still in your torso as you inhale to stretch and exhale to pull.
7. End by pulling both knees into your chest with a deep exhalation and go on to the Single Straight Leg Stretch. . . .

NOTE: Beginners go to the Spine Stretch Forward. . . .

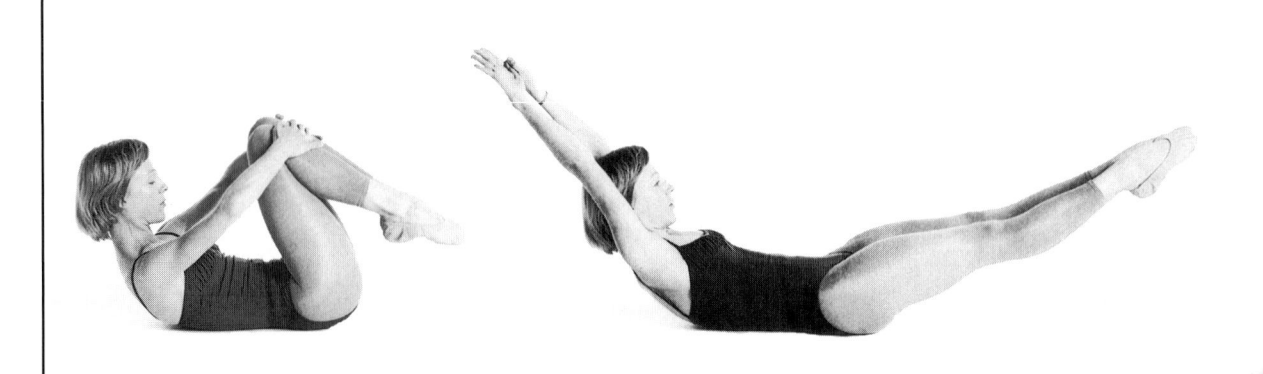

Second of the Stomach Series. Works the powerhouse
and stretches the body.

The Inside Scoop

GOAL
- To remain perfectly still in your torso as you perform the movements.

KEYS
- Support your neck by keeping your chin toward your chest as you stretch long.
- Squeeze your buttocks and upper inner thighs together tightly as you extend your legs to support your lower back.
- As you inhale and stretch out, make sure your arms are straight and feel as if you are being pulled in two directions with only your abdominals to hold you down on the mat.

TIP
- If you press your knees up against your hands and increase the distance between your knees and chest as you exhale, keeping your elbows extended, you will feel a nice release in your upper back and neck area.

NO-NO
- Do not let your head fall back as you stretch your arms above your head.

MODIFICATION
- For a sensitive lower back, straighten your legs to the ceiling instead of to a forty-five-degree angle. As your lower abdominal strength increases, you will be able to begin lowering your legs to a more challenging angle.

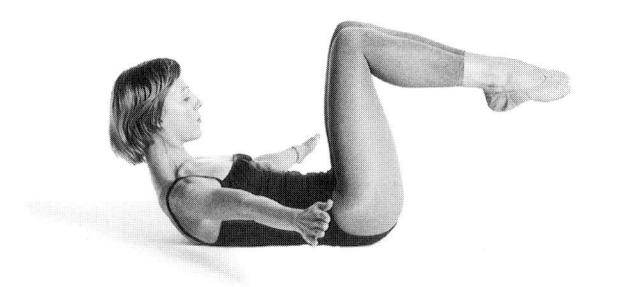

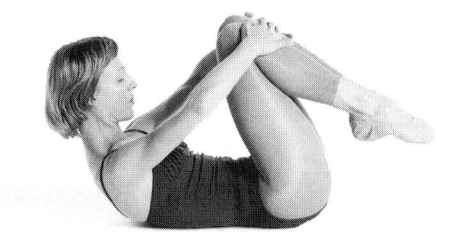

INTERMEDIATE

SINGLE STRAIGHT LEG STRETCH

Step by Step

1. Lie on your back and pull both knees into your chest, elbows extended and head lifted.
2. Extend your right leg straight up to the ceiling and grab your ankle with both hands as you stretch your left leg long in front of you, keeping it hovering slightly above the mat.
3. *Imagine anchoring your torso firmly to the mat* and keep your head lifted onto your chest.
4. Exhale and press your spine deeper into the mat beneath you.
5. Inhale and pull your raised leg in toward your head (keeping it straight) with a double bounce.
6. Exhale and quickly switch the straight legs by scissoring them past each other.
7. Grab the ankle of your left leg and repeat the motion, inhaling for one set and then exhaling for one set. *Imagine the rhythm of windshield wipers beating.*
8. Complete five to ten sets and end by bringing both legs together at a ninety-degree angle in the Pilates stance, and place your hands behind your lifted head to prepare for the Double Straight Leg Stretch. . . .

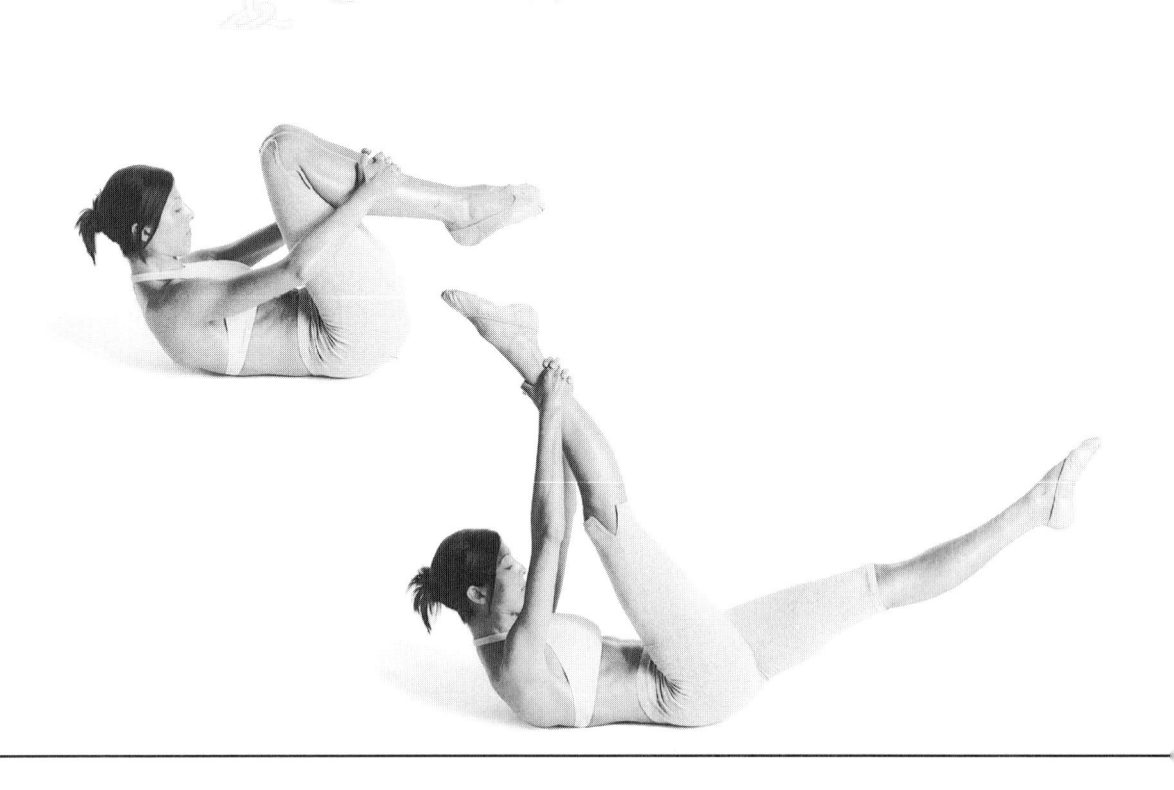

Third of the Stomach Series. Provides for an additional stretch in the back of the legs while still working the abdominal region.

The Inside Scoop

GOAL
- To remain perfectly still in your torso as you stretch and scissor your legs.

KEYS
- Use your sense of rhythm to control the dynamic of this exercise, with small pulses on each stretch.
- Keep your eyes focused on your belly and make sure that it is scooping at all times.

NO-NOS
- Make sure you are not sinking or hunching your shoulders with each beat. Keep lifted from the back of the chest area instead.
- Do not rely on your shoulders to hold the weight of your leg overhead. Use that powerhouse!

BEGINNING
- If this stretch proves too difficult in the beginning, hold lower down on your leg. Try your calf first, and if it is still too difficult, move your hands to the back of your thigh. Do not hold behind your knee.

PROGRESSION
- For a more advanced version, try the exercise with your arms reaching long by your sides. Use control and common sense. If it hurts your neck or lower back, stop.

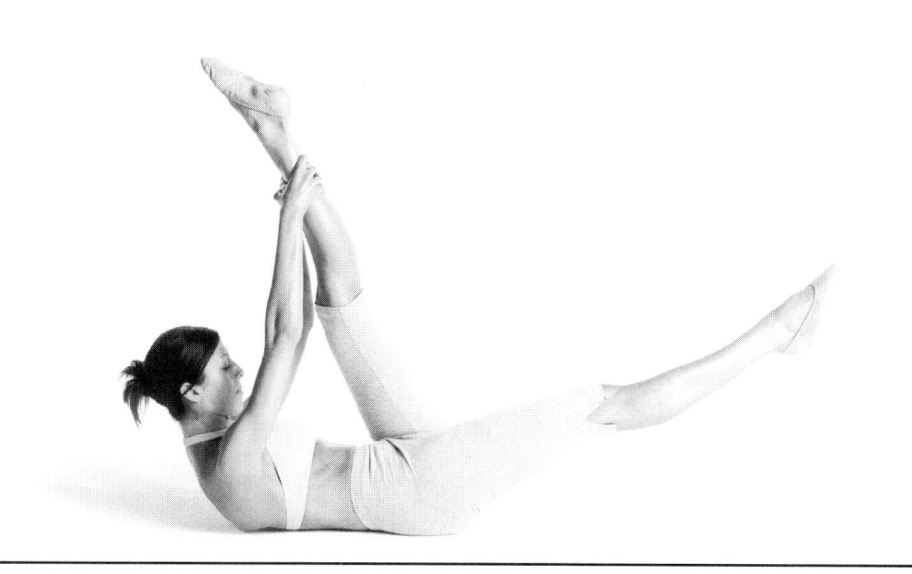

INTERMEDIATE
DOUBLE STRAIGHT LEG STRETCH

Step by Step

1. Lie on your back with your hands, one on top of the other (*not* interlaced), behind your lifted head.
2. Extend your legs straight to the ceiling in the Pilates stance. Squeeze your inner thighs together until no light comes through them.
3. Anchor your center firmly to the mat and lift your head onto your chest. Remember you are lifting from the back of the shoulders and the abdominal muscles, not from the neck, so do not allow your hands to pull the weight of your head forward.
4. Squeeze your buttocks, for stability in your lower back, and lower your straight legs down toward the mat as you inhale. Stop when you feel your lower back begin to arch off the mat.
5. Squeeze your buttocks tighter and exhale as you raise your straight legs toward the ceiling again. You should feel your chest pressing slightly toward the legs as they return to their upright position.
6. *Imagine your legs are attached to springs above your head and you must stretch the springs on the way down and resist their pull on the way back up.*
7. Repeat five to ten times and end by bringing both knees into the chest to prepare for the Crisscross. . . .

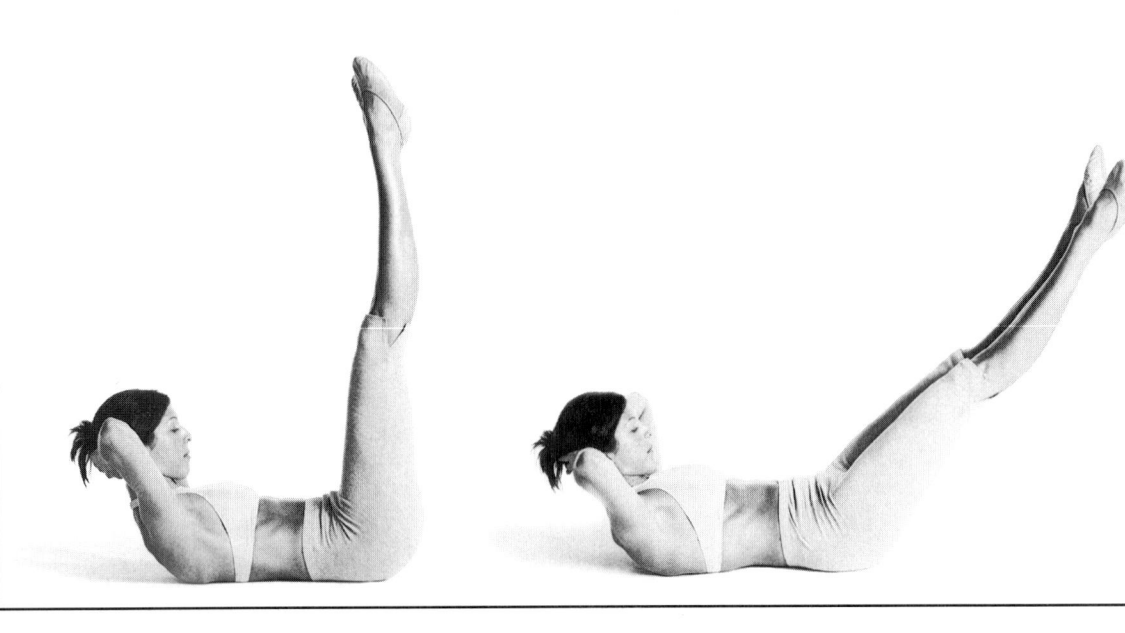

Fourth in the Stomach Series. Targets the powerhouse to the extreme. Upper and lower abdominals help power the stretch up the backs of the legs.

The Inside Scoop

- To remain perfectly still in your torso, with a flat back, as you lower your legs to the floor.
- Keep your elbows extended and press your shoulders down and away from your ears to stretch the muscles of your neck and further increase the focus on the abdominals.
- To accentuate the control element of this movement, keep a slight turnout in the hip and thigh and squeeze extra tight as you bring the legs back up, pressing your chest toward your thighs as you do.
- Make sure you maintain a scooped belly throughout the movement and press your back into the mat beneath you. Feel as though your belly button is lifting and lowering the legs.
- Do not allow your back to arch off the mat as you lower your legs.
- Do not allow your legs or feet to pass your belt line. Stop when they are directly perpendicular to the ceiling.
- In the beginning, and for as long as it serves you, place your hands in a V position just below your tailbone (palms down). This position will help support your lower back.
- For an added challenge, try changing the dynamic of the exercise by switching the accent from the lifting up to the lowering down. (Change the breathing accordingly.)

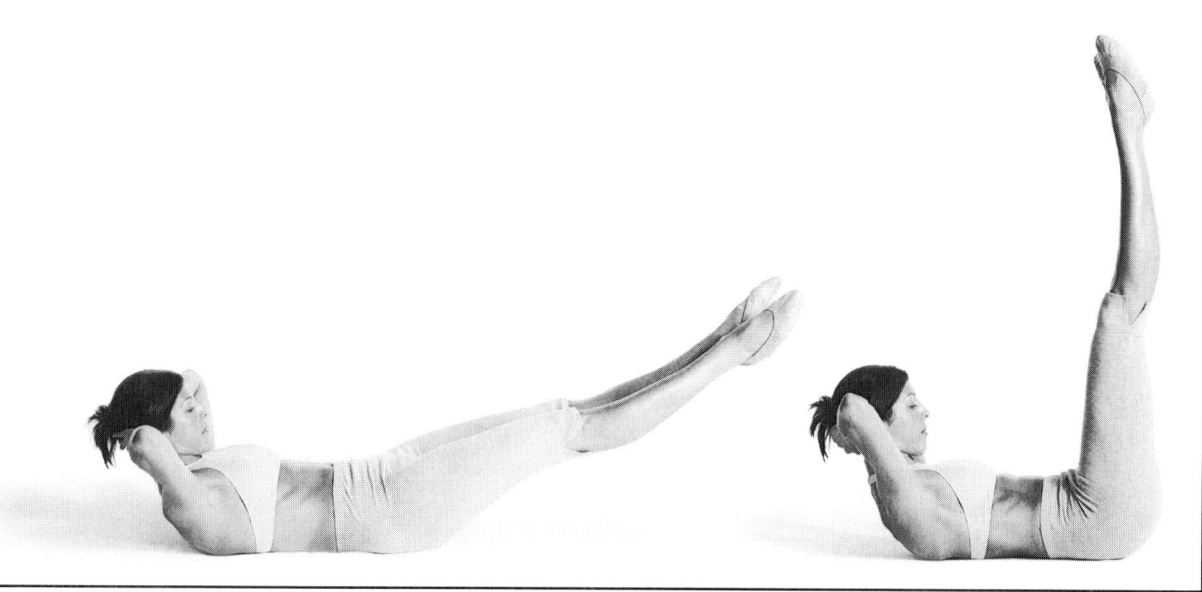

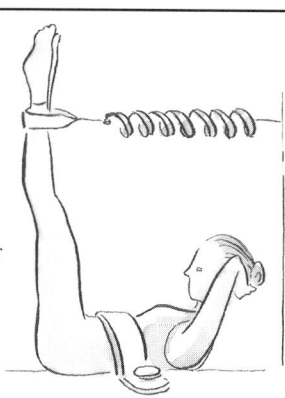

INTERMEDIATE

CRISSCROSS

Step by Step

1. Lie on your back with your hands behind your lifted head and your knees bent into your chest.
2. Extend your right leg out long and above the mat in front of you and twist your upper body until your right elbow touches the left knee. Inhale as you lift to twist.
3. Make sure you are *lifting from below your shoulder* to reach the knee and not simply twisting from the shoulder socket.
4. Look back to your left elbow to increase the stretch and hold the position as you exhale. Make sure your upper back and shoulders do not touch the mat as you twist and hold the stretch.
5. Switch the position by inhaling and bringing your left elbow to your right knee while extending the opposite leg out in front of you. *Hold* the stretch as you exhale completely.
6. *Imagine your center anchored to the mat so that you don't rock from hip to hip.*
7. Complete five to ten sets and then pull your knees tightly into your chest.
8. Roll up to sitting and straighten your legs out in front of you to prepare for the Spine Stretch Forward. . . .

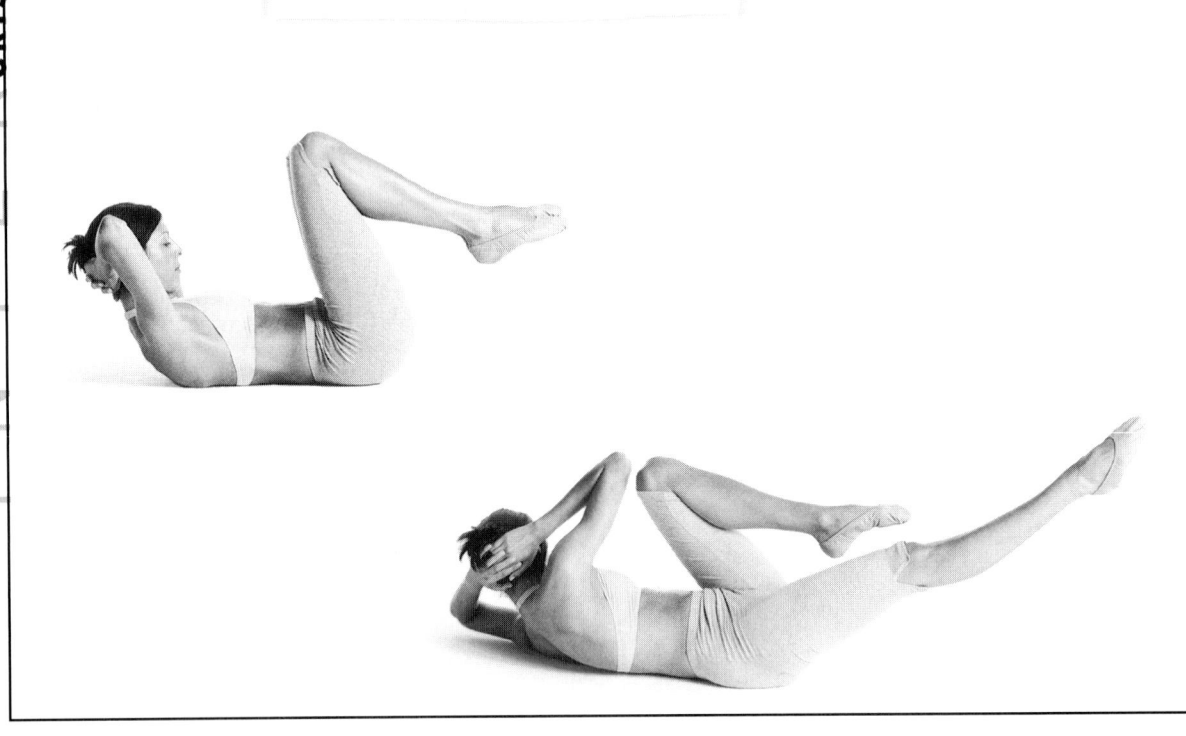

The last of the Stomach Series, the Crisscross works the external obliques, waistline, and powerhouse.

The Inside Scoop

There are many *ways of cheating during this exercise! Here are the major ones.*

- Make sure you are lifting and twisting from your waist and not from your neck and shoulders.
- Keep your elbows extended as much as possible throughout the movements and do not allow them to fold in or to touch the mat as you twist.
- Be sure to actually look back to your elbow as you twist so you can work deeper into your obliques (and even strengthen your ocular muscles).
- Do not rush through this exercise. Really feel the twist and hold the position as you exhale completely.
- Do not allow your outstretched leg to drop too low in front of you. Maintain control by squeezing your buttocks.
- Do not rock your body from side to side as you go. The steadier you remain, the more efficiently you are working.

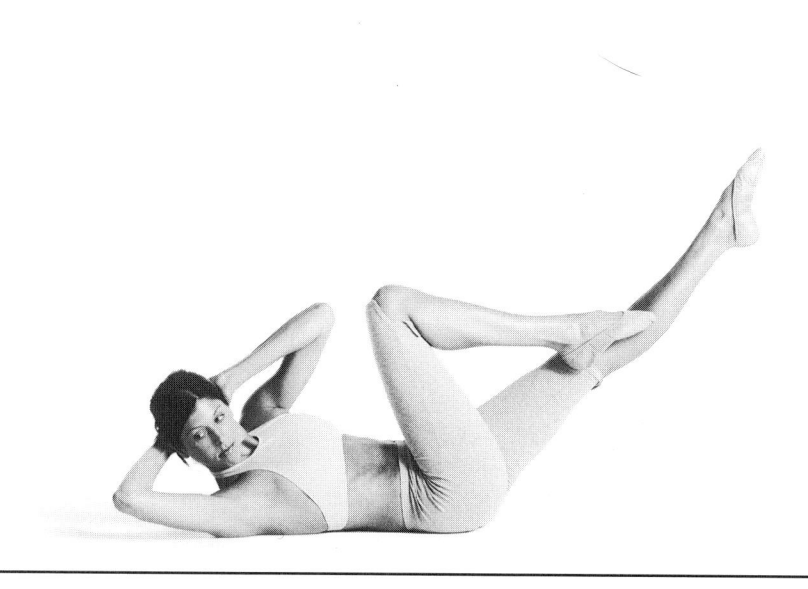

BEGINNER

SPINE STRETCH FORWARD

Step by Step

1. Sit tall with your legs extended straight out on the mat in front of you and open to slightly wider than your hips' width.
2. Straighten your arms out in front of you and flex your feet *as if you were pressing your heels into the wall across the room.*
3. Inhale and sit up even taller as if the crown of your head were pressing up and through the ceiling above.
4. Bring your chin to your chest and begin to round down toward your belly, forcing the air out of your lungs. *Imagine you are forming the letter C with your body.*
5. Exhale as you stretch forward, simultaneously pulling in your abdominals. *Imagine you are stretching over a beach ball held between your legs. Squeeze the imaginary ball with your upper inner thighs* as you lift your chest up over the top.
6. Inhale and reverse the motion of the exercise, *rolling up as if constrained by a wall behind you.*
7. Exhale as you return to your tall seated position, pressing your shoulders down and stretching your arms long in front of you. *Really feel your back stretching flat up against the imagined wall behind you.*
8. Repeat three times with the goal of increasing the stretch down the spine with each repetition. End by sitting tall and bending your knees in toward your chest to prepare for the Open Leg Rocker. . . .

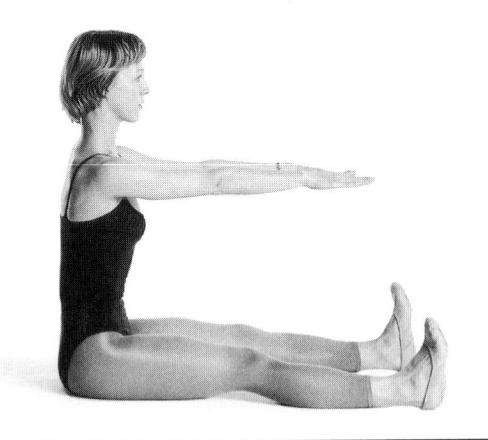

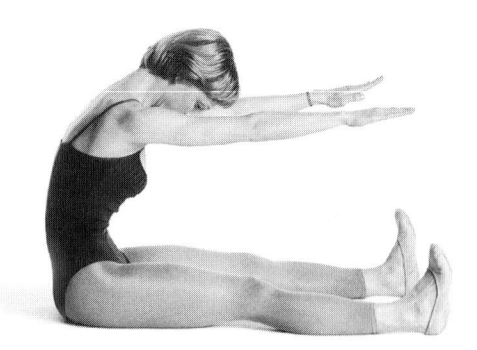

The Spine Stretch Forward articulates the spine and enhances good posture. It also stretches your hamstrings and empties stale air from your lungs.

The Inside Scoop

GOAL
- To keep your hips stable and your belly pulling back as you round and stretch forward.

KEYS
- As you roll up to sitting make sure you are lifting from your powerhouse and not initiating from your head. (Your head should be the last part up.)
- Press your shoulders down and away from your ears as you roll yourself up to release the muscles in the back of your neck. Keep the crown of your head stretching toward the ceiling.
- Think of pulling your baby toes back toward you as you stretch forward.
- Breathe through the stretch to control the movement.
- Try to feel as if you are creating space between each vertebra as you roll up.

NO-NOS
- Do not let your knees roll inward as you stretch forward.
- Roll not back but *up* as you return to your tall seated position.
- Do not hold your breath, as this creates more tension in your body and limits your progress.

PROGRESSION
- As you progress try to increase the stretch by pulling deeper into your spine with each repetition.

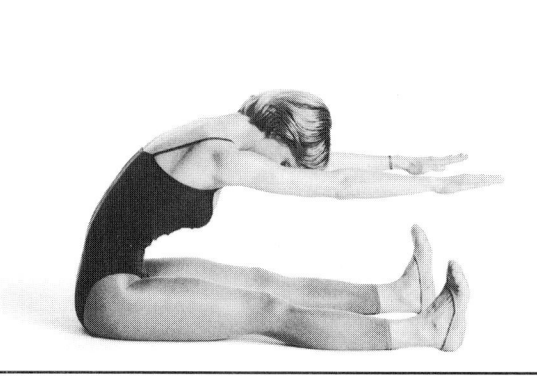

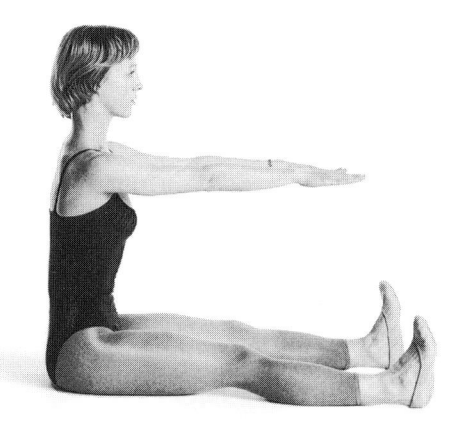

INTERMEDIATE
OPEN-LEG ROCKER

Step by Step

1. Sit toward the front end of your mat with your knees bent in toward your chest. Open your knees to shoulder width and take hold of your ankles.
2. Pull your navel deep into your spine and lean back until you are balancing on your tailbone with your feet off the floor.
3. Straighten both legs toward the ceiling in an open V position and balance. Your arms are straight.
4. To initiate the rocking, inhale, pressing your navel down into your spine, and bring your chin to your chest. Do not initiate the movement by throwing your head back.
5. Roll back just as far as the bottom of your shoulder blades, remaining in your V position, and then exhale to come back up (chin on chest).
6. *Imagine you are sitting in a high-backed rocking chair that is about to tip over, and quickly bring yourself up to a balanced position.*
7. Repeat six times and end by coming up and balancing. Bring your legs together and, leaving them in the air, lay your upper body down onto the mat to prepare for the Corkscrew. . . .

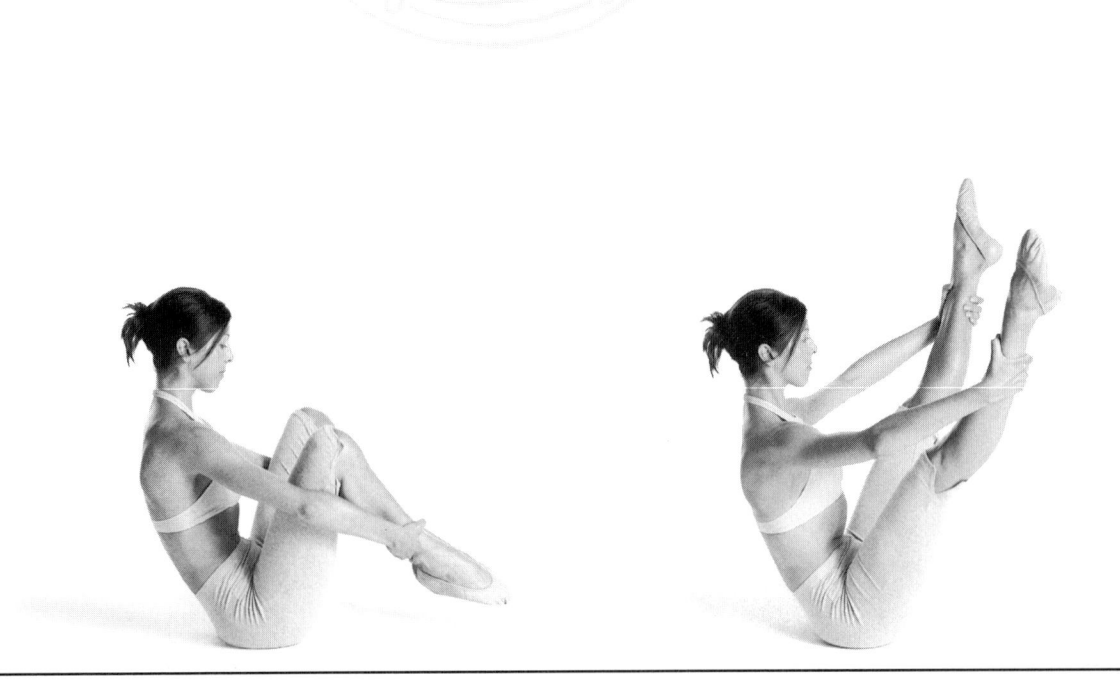

The Open-Leg Rocker massages the spine, stretches your back, works the powerhouse, and is just plain fun!

The Inside Scoop

GOAL
- To be able to hold at your ankles, with straight legs and straight arms, using your powerhouse.

KEYS
- The trick to this exercise is making sure that you are really working from your abdominals and not straining to come up each time. Dynamic is the key.
- Pull in your abdominals to initiate the rocking back, and also to come back up.

NO-NOS
- Do not throw your head back and forth to initiate the movements of this exercise.
- Do not roll onto the back of your neck.

BEGINNING
- Simply try straightening your legs and balancing without rocking. Then try to rock back and up with straight legs, holding behind your calves. (Do not hold behind your knees.)

PROGRESSION
- For an advanced challenge, try placing your hands alongside your ankles (or shins) *without* holding on and rock back and up this way. Do not allow your hands to move from their position. (Remember to initiate from the powerhouse!) Balance at the top of each rocking motion.

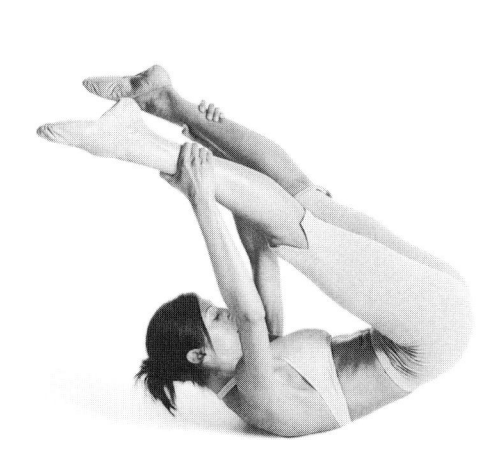

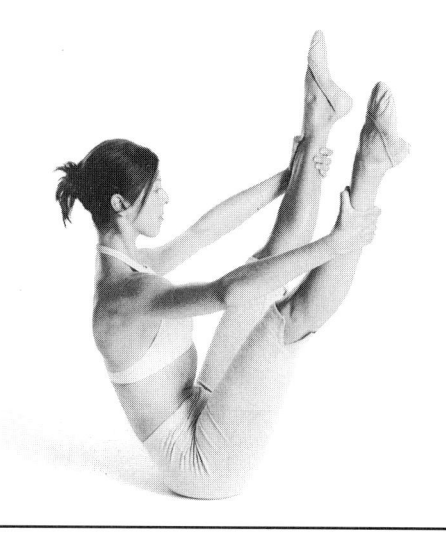

INTERMEDIATE
THE CORKSCREW

Step by Step

1. Lie down on the mat with your legs, in the Pilates stance, extended straight up to the ceiling. Arms are long and heavy by your sides.
2. Inhale and sink your navel to your spine as you circle your legs to the left, down, and around, and then exhale as you bring them back up to their starting position. Do not allow your hips to rock off the mat as you circle your legs. *Imagine your torso is strapped to the mat, leaving only your legs free to move.*
3. Reverse the direction of the circle each time, inhaling as you begin and exhaling as you complete the circle. Your back remains flat against the mat at all times.
4. Make sure to squeeze the buttocks and the upper inner thighs together so that there is no light coming through the legs.
5. Complete three to five sets of the Corkscrew and end by bending your knees into your chest to release your lower back.
6. Roll up to a sitting position with your legs extended on the mat and open slightly wider than your hips' width to prepare for the Saw. . . .

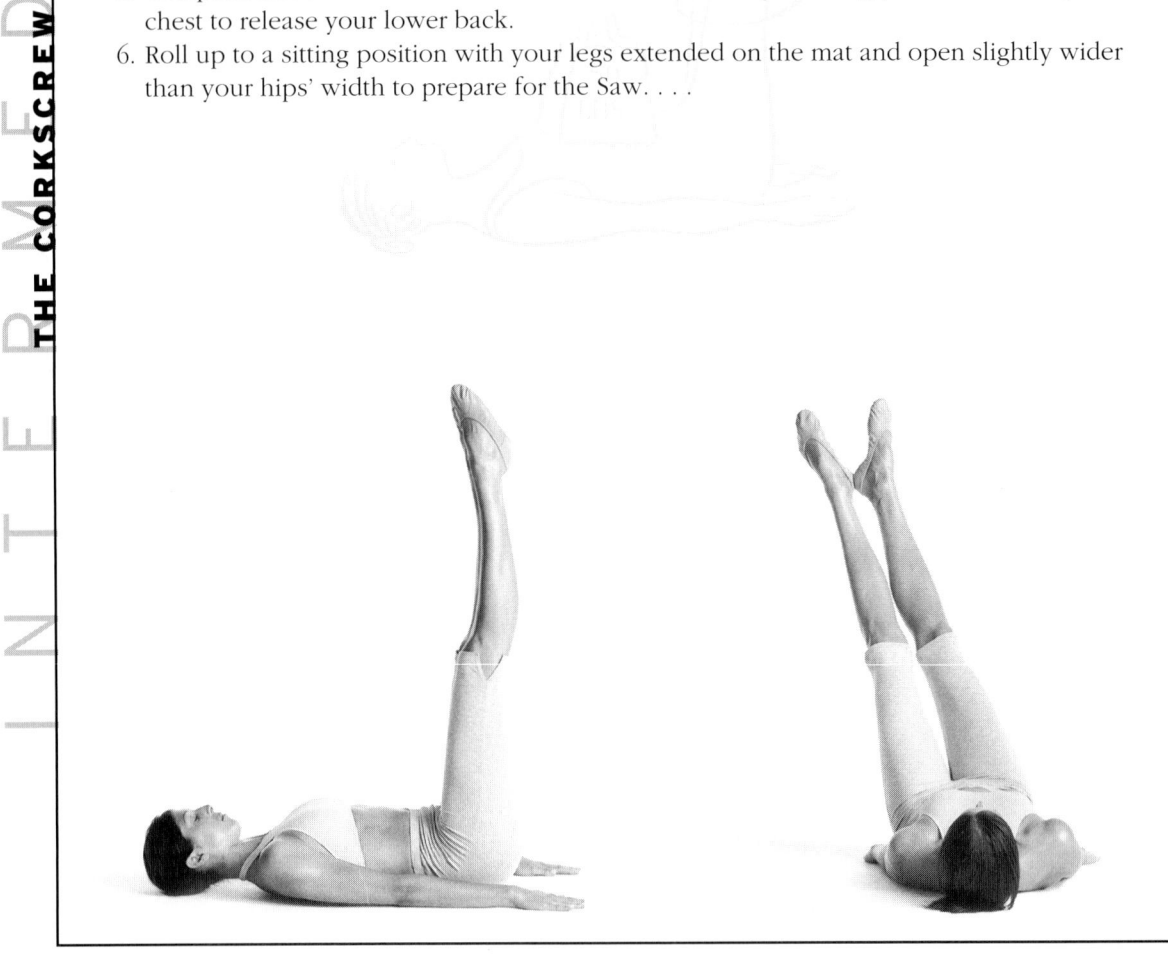

The Corkscrew is meant to target the muscles of the powerhouse, stretch your back, and improve balance.

The Inside Scoop

GOAL
- To keep your neck, back, and shoulders perfectly still and relaxed throughout the movements.

BEGINNING
- Keep the circles very small and tuck your hands in a triangle just below your tailbone to maintain a slight tilt in the hips back toward your center. As your strength and control increase, begin making the circles larger.

KEYS
- Focus on your upper back and shoulders remaining pressed into the mat beneath you.
- Press your palms down into the mat by your sides to stabilize the upper body.
- Scoop your navel down into your spine for support.
- Make sure to squeeze up the back of the inner thighs and buttocks to support your lower back.
- *Imagine your legs have fused together into one.*

NO-NOS
- Do not roll back onto your neck.
- Do not allow your back to arch off the mat.

PROGRESSION
- For the advanced version of this exercise, allow your hips to lift off the mat as you bring your legs back up and over your head, *as if you were drawing a big circle around your entire body in each direction using your feet as your guides.*

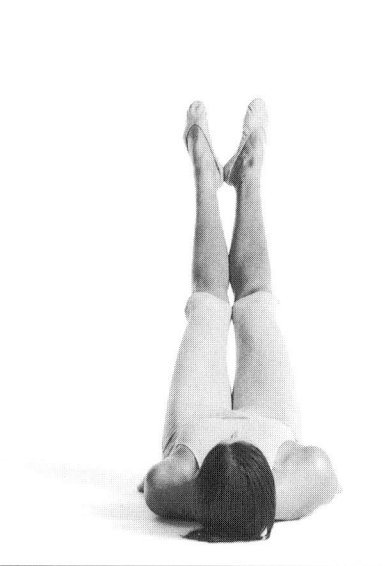

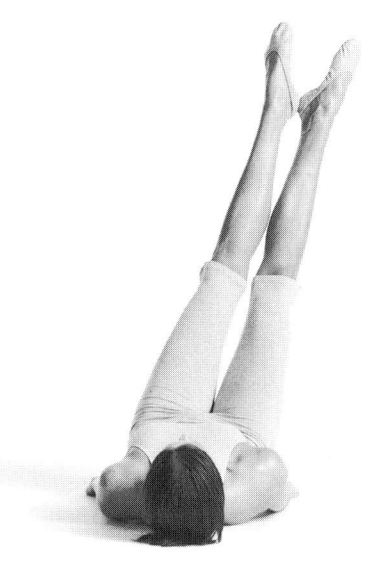

INTERMEDIATE
THE SAW

Step by Step

1. Sit up as tall as possible, with your legs extended and open slightly wider than your hips' width. Flex your feet and push your heels out from under you.
2. Stretch your arms out to your sides as if you were reaching out to touch both sides of the room at once.
3. Inhale and pull your navel up and into your spine, imagining you are stretching the crown of your head up and through the ceiling above.
4. Twist from your waist to the left. Make sure your opposite hip remains pressing down into the mat beneath you. *Imagine you are sitting in a block of cement and are able to move only from just above your hips.*
5. Bring your head and chest toward your right leg, stretching your left arm forward and just past your baby toe. Allow your pinkie finger to brush by the baby toe as if it were a saw.
6. Continue to stretch your chest to the thigh as you deepen the exhalation. Feel your opposite hip deeply imbedded in the cement and unable to move. Stretch the crown of your head toward the baby toe and lift your back arm in opposition.
7. Inhale and draw your body up, initiating from the navel, into the starting position.
8. Repeat the sequence to the right, exhaling deeply as you stretch your head and chest toward the left leg.
9. Complete four sets and then flip onto your stomach to prepare for the Swan Dive....

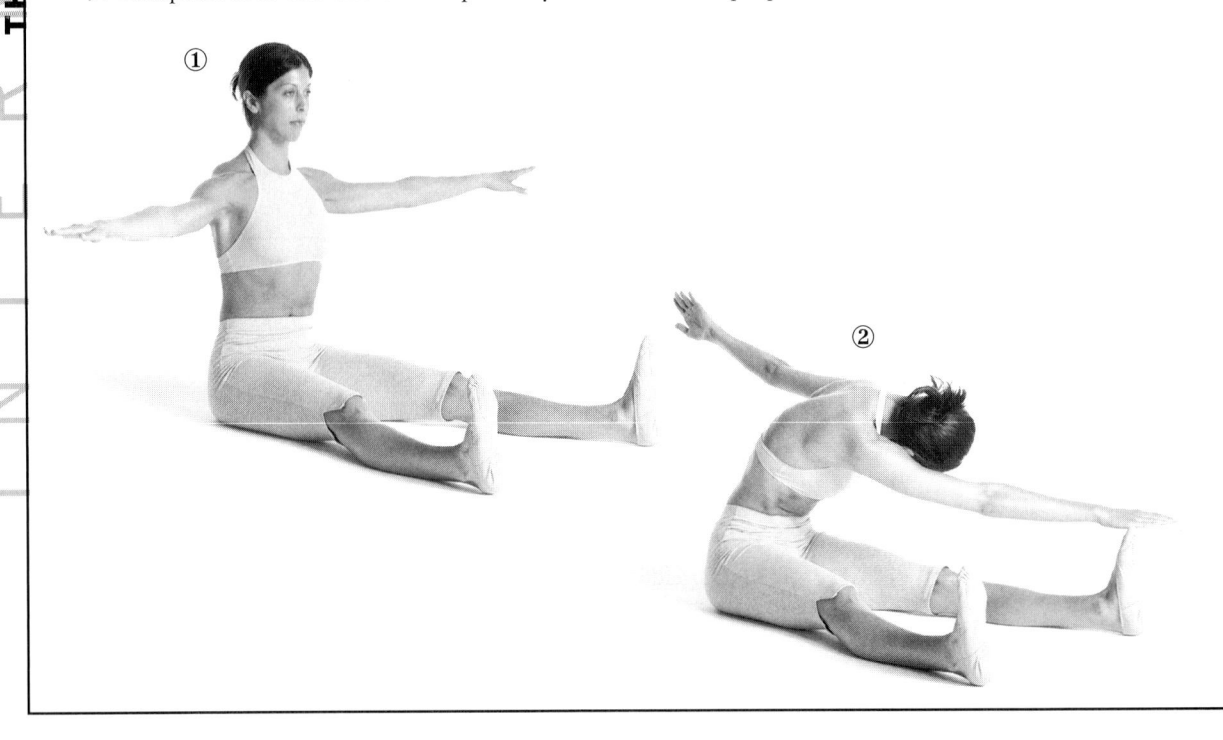

The Saw is a breathing exercise that wrings the stale air from the bottom of your lungs. It works the waistline and stretches the hamstrings.

The Inside Scoop

GOAL

- To keep your hips absolutely still as you stretch past your baby toe, with straight legs and back arm lifted.

KEYS

- Stabilize your hips as you stretch in each direction. Think of pressing your opposite heel forward and sitting on the opposite buttock as you stretch.
- Roll up to a tall seated position and inhale before twisting to the other side. Think of filling your lungs with air and then wringing them out as you twist on the exhalation.
- Once again, initiate coming up from the powerhouse (abdominals and buttocks). Your head should be the last part to come up. (Remember to sit up, not back.)

NO-NOS

- Do not scrunch up in your neck as you reach past your baby toe. Lengthen from the crown of the head instead.
- Do not allow your knees to roll in as you stretch forward.

MODIFICATION

- If this stretch proves too difficult, simply soften the opposite knee, or both knees if necessary. As your flexibility increases, begin keeping both legs absolutely straight throughout.

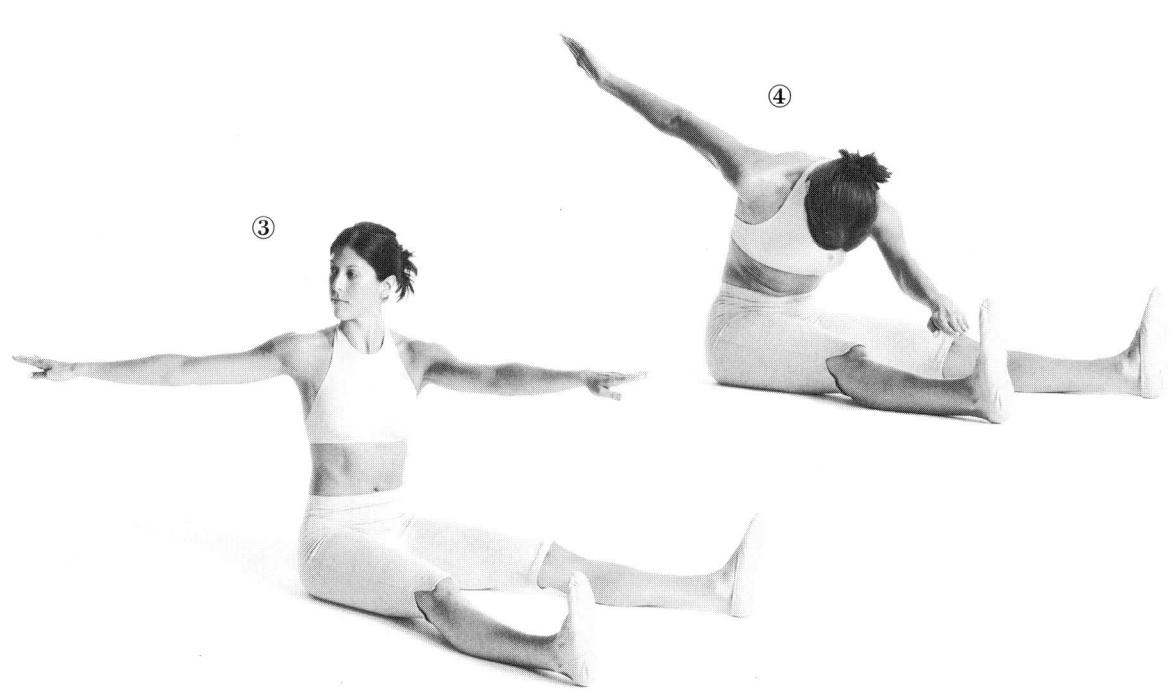

ADVANCED
SWAN DIVE

Step by Step

1. Lie on your stomach with your palms pressing into the mat directly beneath your shoulders. Squeeze your legs together tightly and allow the tops of your feet to press into the mat behind you.
2. As you inhale, draw your navel up into your spine and begin straightening your arms. Keep your chest lifting and your neck long. (Do not drop your head back.)
3. Exhale and bend your arms, lowering yourself back down to the mat. Keep squeezing the buttocks and upper inner thighs together to support your lower back.
4. Do this stretch two or three times to warm up your back muscles for the Swan Dive. . . .

   NOTE: If you are at an intermediate level, go on to the Single Leg Kicks. . . .

5. On the last stretch upward, with your chest reaching for the ceiling, release your hands and inhale, rocking forward onto your breastbone with your arms extended in front of you, palms up, and your straight legs lifted behind you. *Imagine that you are diving forward to catch a beach ball.*
6. With the same momentum, exhale and rock back, lifting in your chest, and *imagine throwing the ball back over your head.* (Keep arms and legs straight throughout the rocking motion.)
7. Keep rocking back and forth, inhaling forward and exhaling back.
8. Rock for a maximum of five Swan Dives and then sit onto your heels with your forehead on the mat to release your lower back.
9. Hold this rest position for one or two breaths and then lie on your stomach, propped up on your elbows, to go on to the Single Leg Kicks. . . .

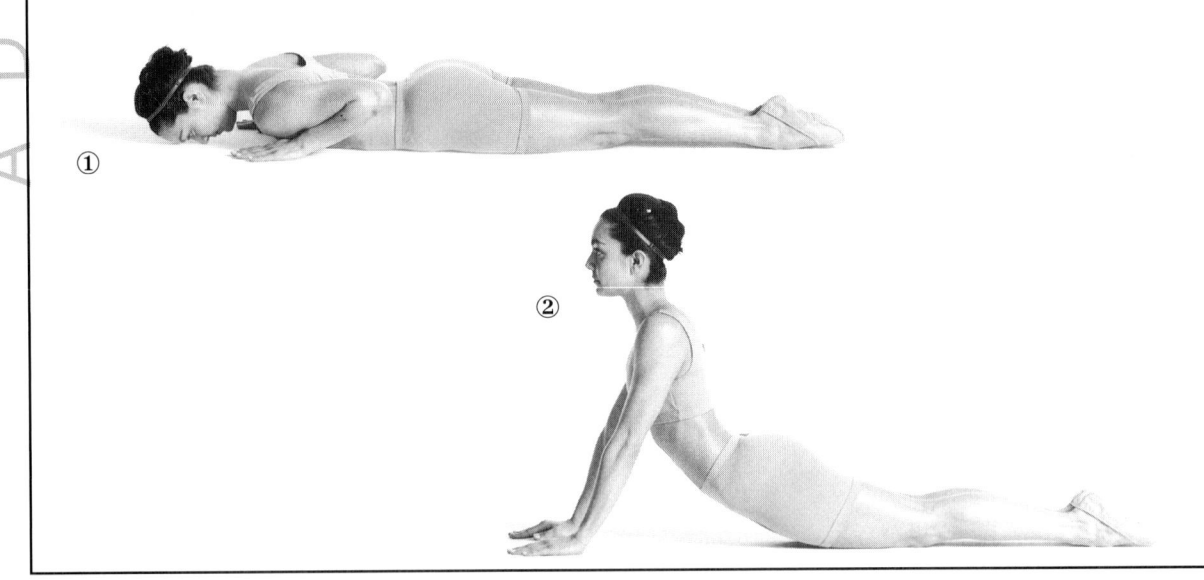

①

②

The Swan Dive stretches and strengthens all the muscles of the back, neck, and shoulders.

The Inside Scoop

If you have a bad back leave this exercise out. Make your goal slowly building up to the preparation stretch only.

- To maintain a rigid body as you rock with your legs glued together and arms straight.
- Breathing and dynamic are the keys to this exercise. Keep the momentum going and focus on your breath throughout.
- Remember to engage the muscles of your powerhouse throughout the Swan Dive to protect the sensitive muscles that run along the spine. It does not take very much to strain these muscles, and once you do, the ache is hard to overcome. Listen to your body. If it hurts, stop.
- Keep your heels together for the entire Swan Dive. If this proves too difficult, allow them to separate slightly, but do not release the muscles of the buttocks.
- Do not throw your head back and forth as you go. Lift from your chest and lengthen the back of your neck to secure the weight of your head.

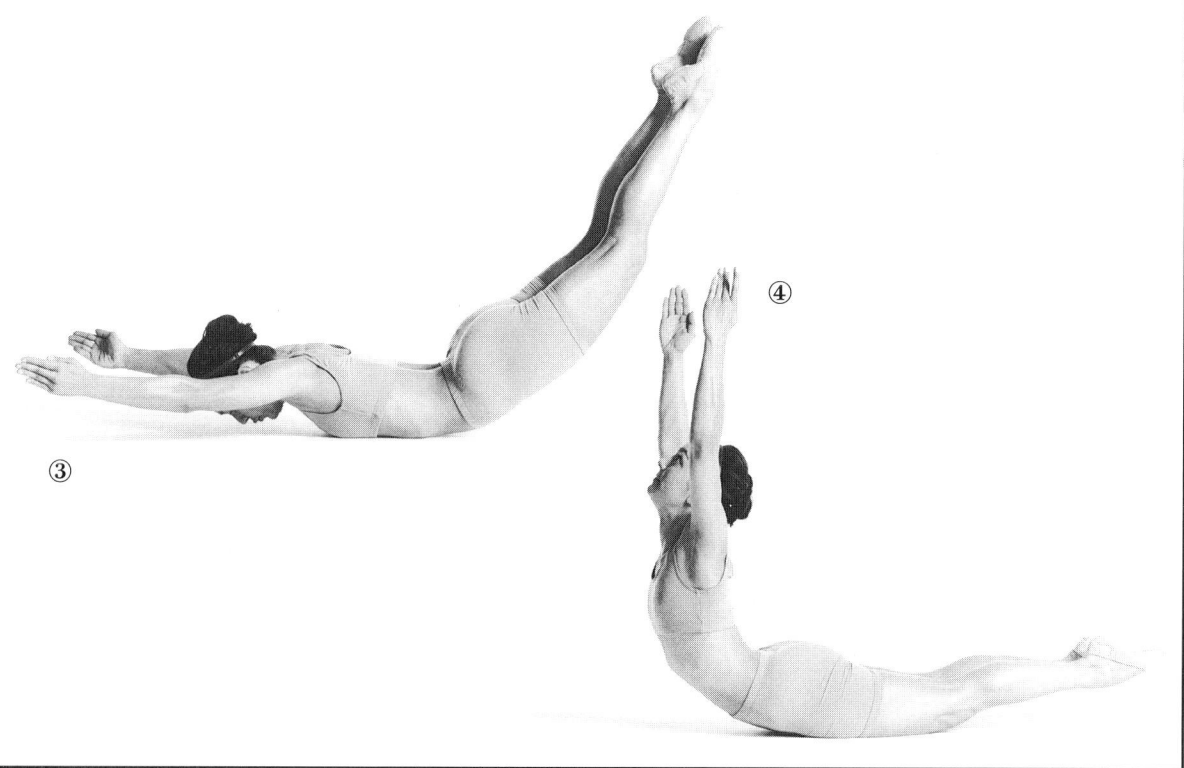

INTERMEDIATE

SINGLE LEG KICKS

Step by Step

1. Lie on your stomach, propped up on your elbows, with your navel pulled up into your spine and your pubic bone pressing firmly down into the mat.
2. Squeeze your buttocks and the backs of your upper inner thighs together to support your lower back. Make sure that your elbows are *directly* beneath your shoulders and your chest is lifted so that you do not sink into your shoulders and back of the neck.
3. Your hands can be made into fists and positioned directly in front of your elbows. (If fists are uncomfortable, place your palms facedown on the mat.) Think of lifting your upper body away from the mat by pressing away from the elbows.
4. *Imagine you are being suspended from the ceiling from your belly and must continue to press your elbows and pelvic bone into the mat to stay grounded.*
5. Lengthen your spine and kick your left heel into your left buttock with a double beat.
6. Switch and kick the right heel to the right buttock with a double beat. Straighten the opposite leg when it is not kicking. Do not let it touch the mat in between kicks.
7. Remember to stay lifted in the abdominals by pressing up and away from your elbows.
8. Complete five sets and end by sitting back on your heels to release your lower back. Lie onto your stomach with your face to one side and your hands behind your back to prepare for the Double Leg Kicks. . . .

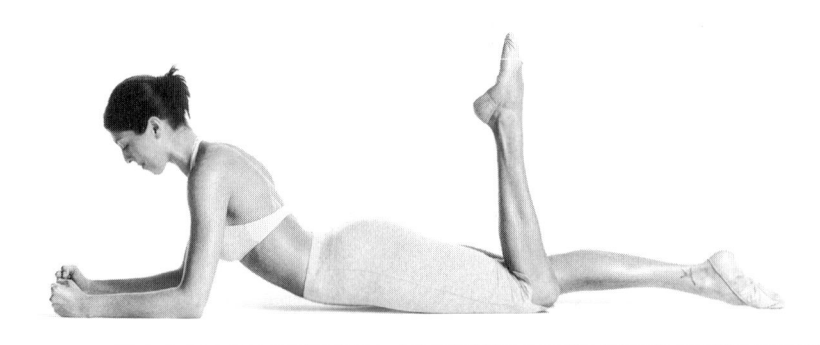

The Single Leg Kicks work your hamstrings, biceps, and triceps while stretching your thighs, knees, and abdominal muscles.

The Inside Scoop

If you have bad knees, leave this exercise out, or simply use the motion of slowly bringing your heel toward your buttock as a stretch over the knee. If you experience pain, stop.

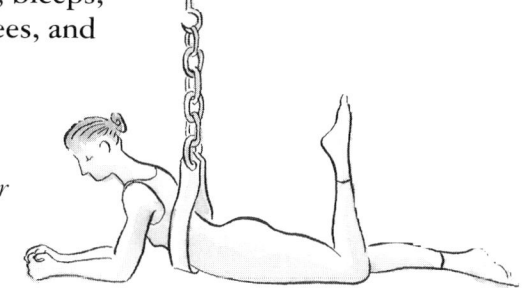

- To remain lifted and perfectly still in your torso as you kick your heels into your bottom.
- The key to this exercise is maintaining a lifted upper body throughout the kicking movement. This is best achieved by lifting your chest up and away from your elbows while still pressing your pubic bone into the mat.
- Make sure to lengthen from the crown of your head to maintain a long neck and to support the weight of your head.
- Keep your upper thighs and knees glued together as you kick to engage the hamstring and buttock muscles.
- Do not sink into your shoulders or lower back.
- If your lower back hurts, stop. Sit back on your heels and release your back.

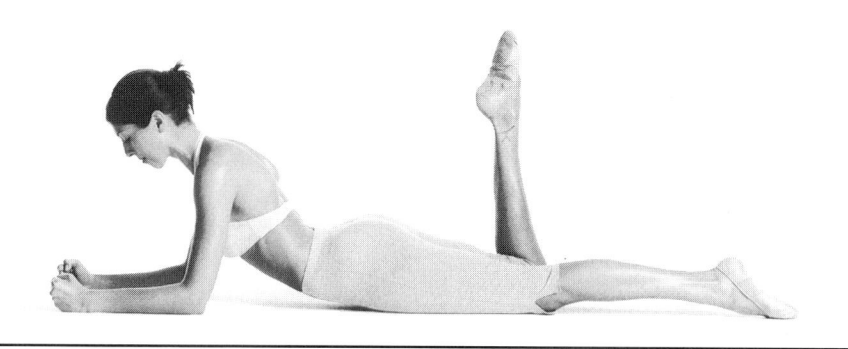

INTERMEDIATE
DOUBLE LEG KICKS

Step by Step

1. Lie on your stomach with your face resting on one side. Clasp your hands behind you and place them as high up on your back as is comfortable while still being able to touch the fronts of your shoulders and elbows down to the mat.
2. Squeeze your buttocks and upper inner thighs together and inhale as you kick both heels, *like a fish's tail,* to your bottom three times.
3. As you extend your legs back down to the mat, exhale and stretch your arms back to follow them, bringing your upper back up off the mat in an arched position.
4. Continue to reach your clasped hands long and low behind you, squeezing your shoulder blades together and lengthening your spine. Keep your legs and the tops of your feet pressing down into the mat beneath you as you stretch back.
5. Exhale as you return your upper body to the mat, turning your face to the other side and bringing your hands and heels back to the initial kicking position.
6. *Imagine your hands and feet are connected by a band that is pulled back and forth between them.*
7. Complete three sets of the Double Leg Kicks and then sit back onto your heels to release the lower back. Flip onto your back and lie with your hands behind your head and your legs outstretched on the mat to prepare for the Neck Pull. . . .

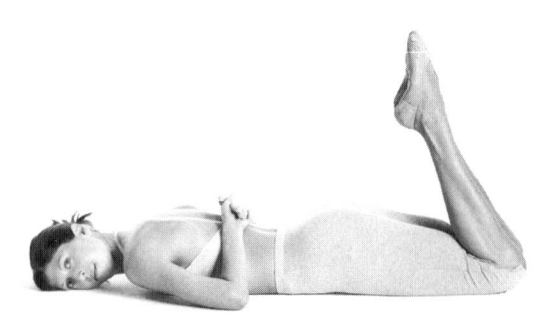

The Double Leg Kicks work the back of the legs and buttocks and stretch the shoulders and midback.

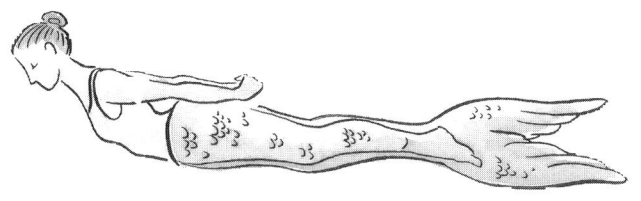

The Inside Scoop

If you have a bad back or shoulders, leave this exercise out.

G·O·A·L
- To be able to touch your heels to your buttocks during the kicks. To press your elbows into the mat with your hands high on your back. To keep your legs together and your feet down when stretching your back.

K·E·Y·S
- Make sure to keep your arms reaching long and low behind you. Think of trying to get your hands down past your buttocks.
- Keep the tops of your feet pressing into the mat as you stretch back, engaging the muscles of the buttocks and thighs throughout.
- Make sure you are pulling your navel up into your spine throughout to support your lower back.
- If you feel pain in your back, stop! Sit back onto your heels with your arms outstretched and release your upper and lower back.

N·O–N·O·S
- Do not allow your head to sink back into your shoulders. Lengthen the back of your neck by pressing forward and up from the crown of the head, keeping your chest lifted.
- Do not allow your buttocks to lift up as you kick your heels into them.

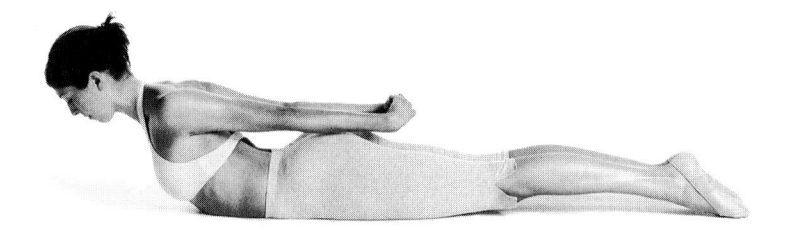

INTERMEDIATE
NECK PULL

Step by Step

1. Lie on your back with your hands, one on top of the other, behind the base of your head.
2. Extend your legs straight out on the mat and open them to your hips' width. Flex your feet and glue your heels to the mat. Make sure your back is flat and your navel is pressing down into your spine.
3. Inhale and begin rolling up and forward, squeezing your buttocks to initiate the movement. Remember the sequence to rolling up: Lift your chin to your chest, lift your chest up over your ribs, lift your ribs up over your belly, then try to lift your belly up and over your hips. Think of peeling yourself up off the mat and curling forward.
4. *Imagine your legs are strapped to the mat just below your hips.*
5. Exhale as you round your back over your thighs as if taking a bow. Keep your elbows wide and your legs firmly anchored to the mat.
6. Inhale and draw yourself up to a tall seated position *as if pressing up against an imaginary wall behind you.* Remember to lift up and not back.
7. Exhale as you slightly tuck your tailbone underneath you and begin slowly rolling your spine back down to the mat. Try to feel each vertebra stretching down to the mat, as if you were putting a space between each one.
8. Repeat the Neck Pull five times and end by lying on your back with your knees bent in toward your chest to prepare for the Scissors. . . .

   NOTE: If you are not advanced, or if you have any sign of a weak back, do not perform the next five exercises. End the Neck Pull instead by lying on your side, and go on to the Side Kick Series (p. 98). . . .

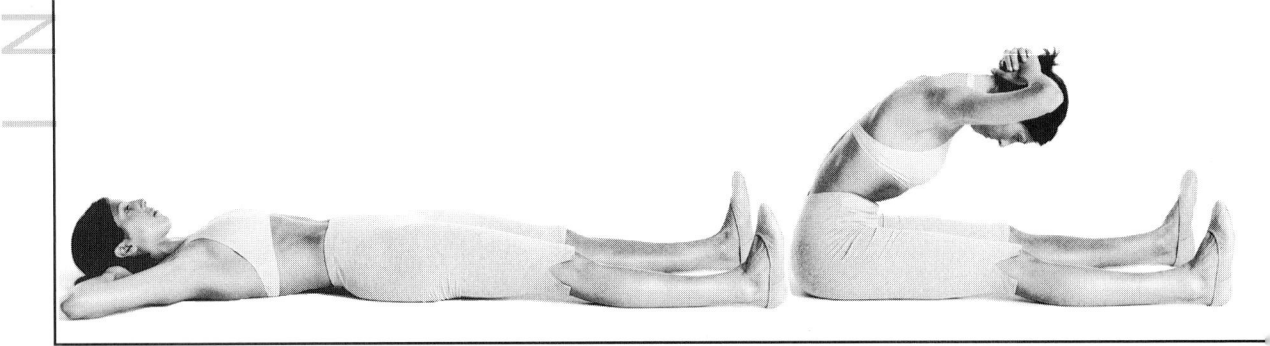

The Neck Pull strengthens your powerhouse, stretches your hamstrings, articulates your spine, and improves posture.

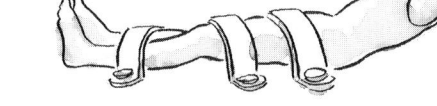

The Inside Scoop

GOAL
- To keep your legs glued to the mat at all times, not letting them slide forward or back.

KEYS
- The key to the Neck Pull is remaining fixed in the lower body as you perform the sequence. *Imagine your feet are two lead weights that cannot be budged. Your legs are the rods that hold them in place.*
- Keep your elbows outstretched throughout the movements.
- Initiate the movements from deep within the abdominals and engage your powerhouse throughout.
- Articulate your spine as you peel yourself off the mat and press each vertebra into the mat on the way down.

NO-NO
- Do not pull forward so hard on your head as to strain the muscles in the back of your neck.

MODIFICATION
- If you are unable to come up with straight legs, bend your knees and use your hands to "walk" up the underside of your thighs. Stretch forward, straightening your legs and placing your hands behind your head. Roll up to a tall seated position and then, bending your knees and replacing your hands on the underside of your thighs, lower yourself back down, pressing each vertebra into the mat as you go.

PROGRESSION
- For an advanced variation, try to keep your upper body more rigid, lengthening as you roll back. Still touch each vertebra down to the mat as you go.

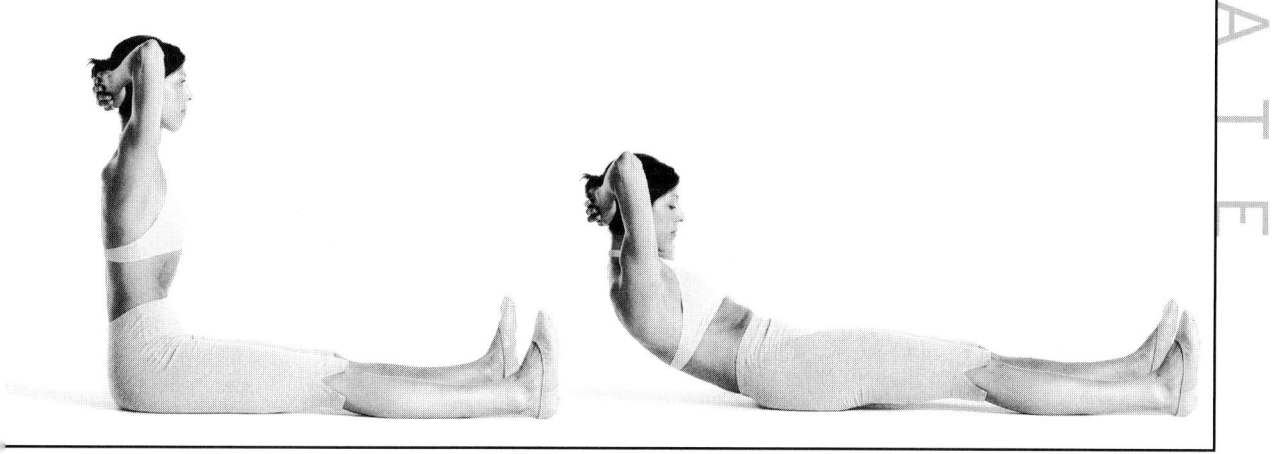

VERY ADVANCED

THE SCISSORS

Step by Step

1. Lie flat on your mat with your legs straight and feet long.
2. Bring your legs straight up to a ninety-degree angle, and continue lifting by pressing your hips and legs up to the ceiling.
3. Place your hands on your back, just above your hips, so that you are stabilized in a lifted position.
4. Pull your navel deep into your spine and squeeze your buttocks tightly to secure your position.
5. Inhale and reach one leg long toward the mat while the other reaches over your head in a splitlike movement.
6. Allow your legs to pulse slightly without wobbling in your base.
7. Switch legs by scissoring them past each other and exhale as your opposite leg now pulses overhead.
8. Complete three sets of Scissors and remain in a lifted position to prepare for the Bicycle. . . .

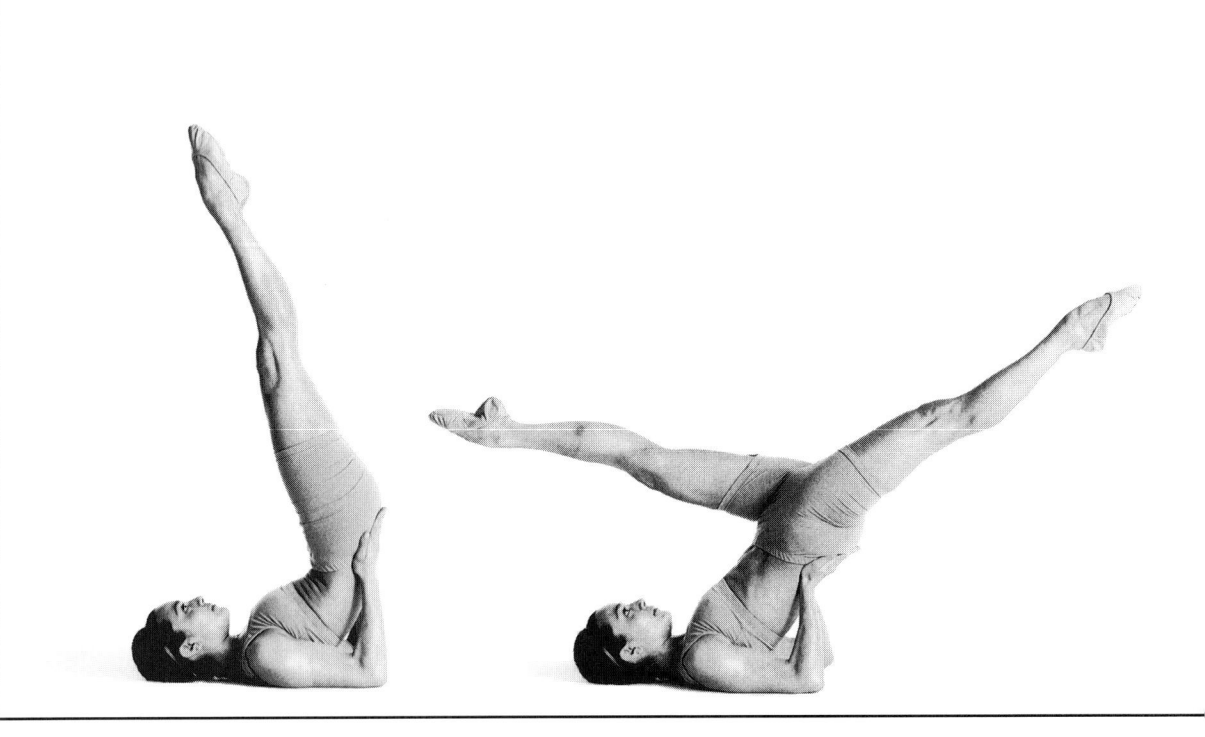

The Scissors stretch your hip flexors, quads, and hamstrings while building strength in the powerhouse and increasing the flexibility of your spine.

The Inside Scoop

Do not perform the Scissors and the Bicycle if you have a bad neck, shoulder, or wrist.

- To remain stable and controlled in your hips while allowing your legs to scissor into alternating straight-legged splits.

- Keep lifting in your hips.
- Use your buttocks and abdominals to provide the strength necessary for this movement.
- To increase the stretch, think of reaching your ankles as far away from each other as possible as you pulse.
- Focus on the forward leg reaching away from you so that you do not sink into your neck and shoulders.
- Breathe!

- Do not allow the weight of your body to rest solely on your neck and/or hands.
- Do not allow your knees to bend as you go. Stretch only as far as is possible with straight legs.

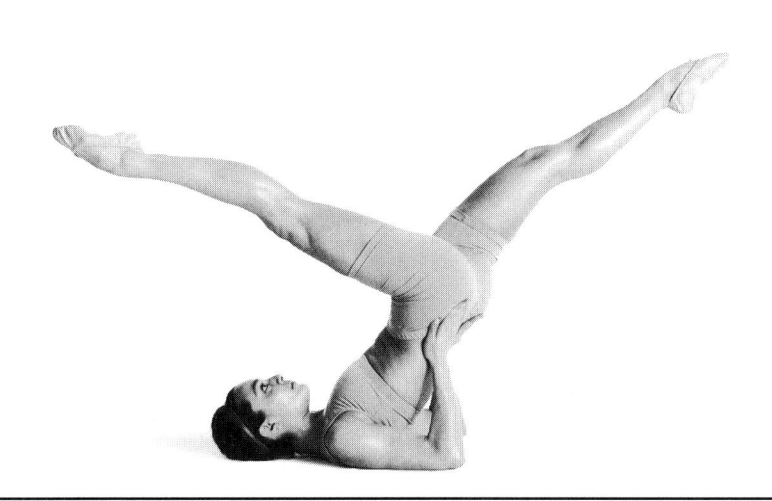

VERY ADVANCED
THE BICYCLE

Step by Step

1. Remain in the lifted position from the Scissors and adjust your hands so you are holding your hips steady.
2. Reach your left leg to the ceiling as you stretch your right leg down toward the mat in front of you.
3. Bend your right knee and draw your heel in toward your bottom.
4. As you bring your right knee in toward your chest, allow your left leg to stretch down toward the mat in front of you.
5. Repeat the sequence with your left leg and then continue "pedaling" for three sets.
6. *Imagine you are trying to keep your feet on the pedals of a big bicycle as you go.*
7. After three sets forward, reverse the pedaling movement and complete three sets in reverse.
8. End by allowing your back to roll down to the mat and place the soles of your feet flat on the floor to prepare for the Shoulder Bridge. . . .

NOTE: For an advanced transition to the Shoulder Bridge, finish the Bicycle by lowering the soles of your feet slowly down to the mat with your back still propped up on your hands. Change your support position by turning your hands to the outside and grasping the undersides of your hip bones.

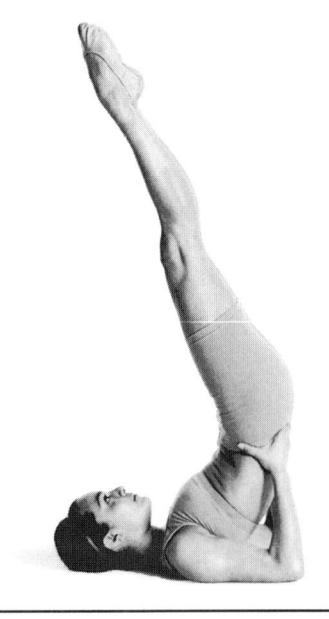

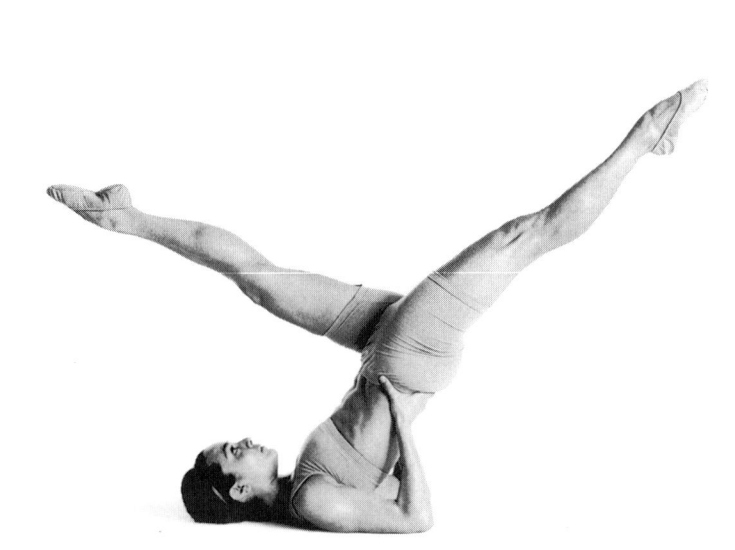

The Bicycle works the backs of your legs while simultaneously stretching your hips and thighs.

The Inside Scoop

If you have a bad back, neck, wrist, or shoulder, leave this exercise out.

GOALS
- To remain perfectly still and lifted in your hips as you perform the cycling movements.
- The accent is on reaching each leg forward and trying to touch your toe to the floor as you "pedal."

KEYS
- Keep your navel pressed to your spine throughout.
- *Imagine you are glued to your hands.*
- Use your powerhouse to control the movements.

NO-NOS
- Do not sink into your wrists.
- Do not arch your lower back to the point where your belly sticks out.

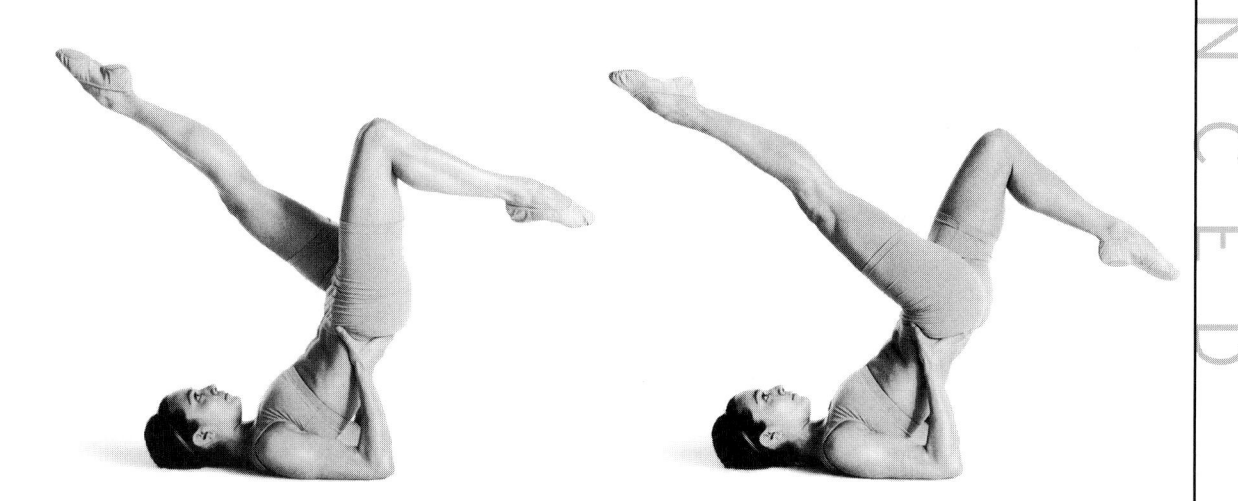

VERY ADVANCED
SHOULDER BRIDGE

Step by Step

1. If you have not made the advanced transition from The Bicycle then lie on your back with your knees bent, hips' width apart, and the soles of your feet planted firmly on the mat.
2. Squeeze your buttocks up off the mat and raise your hips until you are able to place a hand under the back of each hip. Your elbows are directly under each hand and your fingers face outward. *Imagine you are suspended from the ceiling by a sling around your hips.*
3. Pull your navel deep into your spine and secure the muscles of your powerhouse.
4. Stretch one leg out long in front of you and kick it up to the ceiling, inhaling as you go.
5. Flex your foot at the highest point and, exhaling, lower your leg, stretching it long out of your hip as it goes.
6. Perform three to five kicks and return your foot to its original position on the mat.
7. Repeat the sequence with your other leg and then remove your hands, slowly rolling your back down onto the mat. Pull your knees into your chest to release the muscles of your lower back and then sit tall with your legs outstretched to prepare for the Spine Twist. . . .

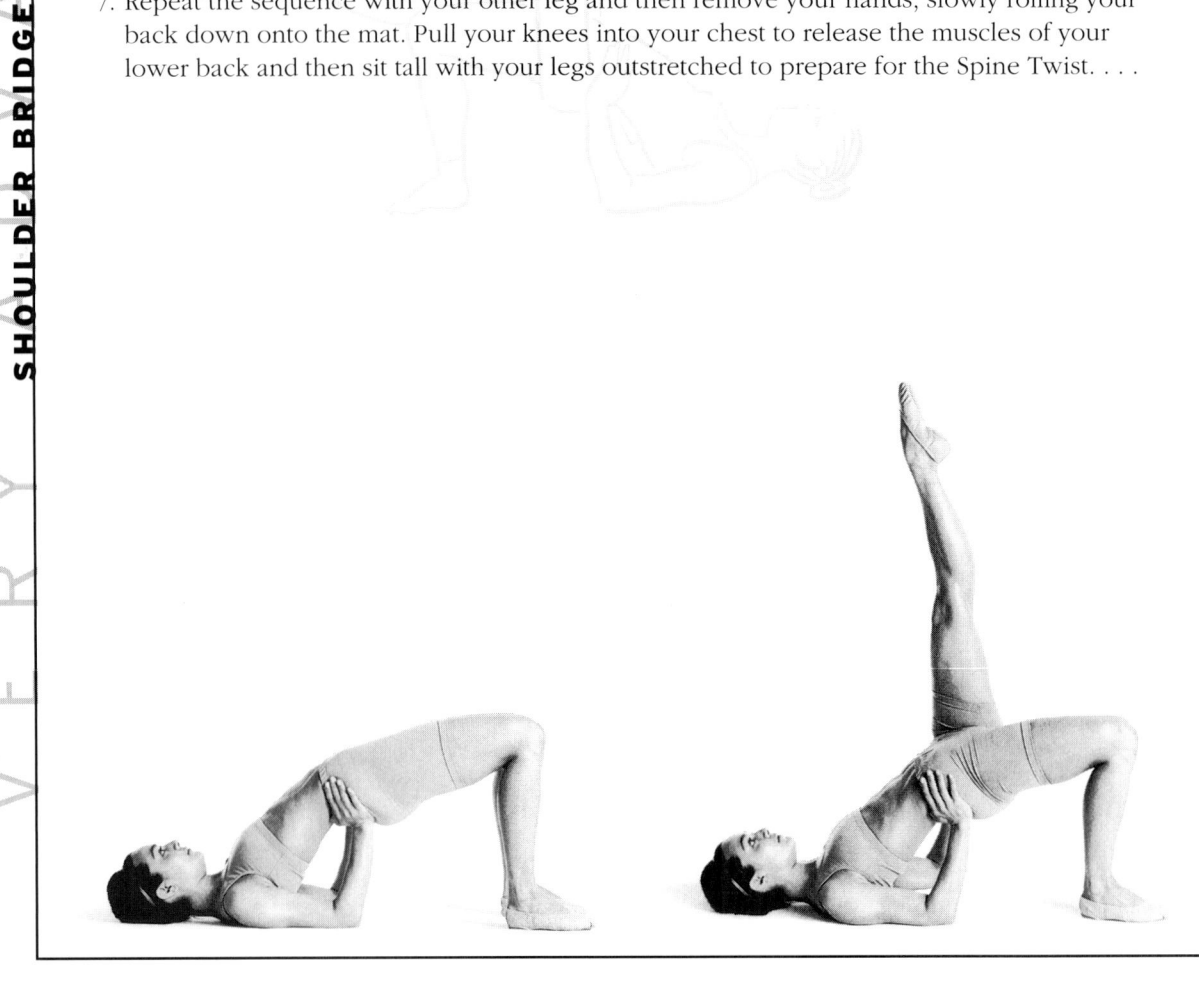

The Shoulder Bridge works the powerhouse, the thighs, and the backs of the legs.

The Inside Scoop

If you have a bad back, wrist, knee, or elbow, leave this exercise out.

GOAL
- To remain perfectly still and lifted in your hips as you perform the leg sequence.

KEYS
- Keep your navel pressed to your spine and squeeze your buttocks throughout.
- Kick only to the highest point you can manage without dropping in your back.
- Keep stretching long out of your hips as you lower and lift your leg (without arching or sinking in your back).
- Stay lifted in your hips by pressing into the standing leg to maintain balance and control.
- Keep your leg aligned with your hip throughout the kicking sequence.

NO-NOS
- Do not sink your weight into your hands or neck.
- Do not allow your leg to drop to the mat as you lower it.

PROGRESSION
- You can add a double kick at the top before slowly lowering your leg.

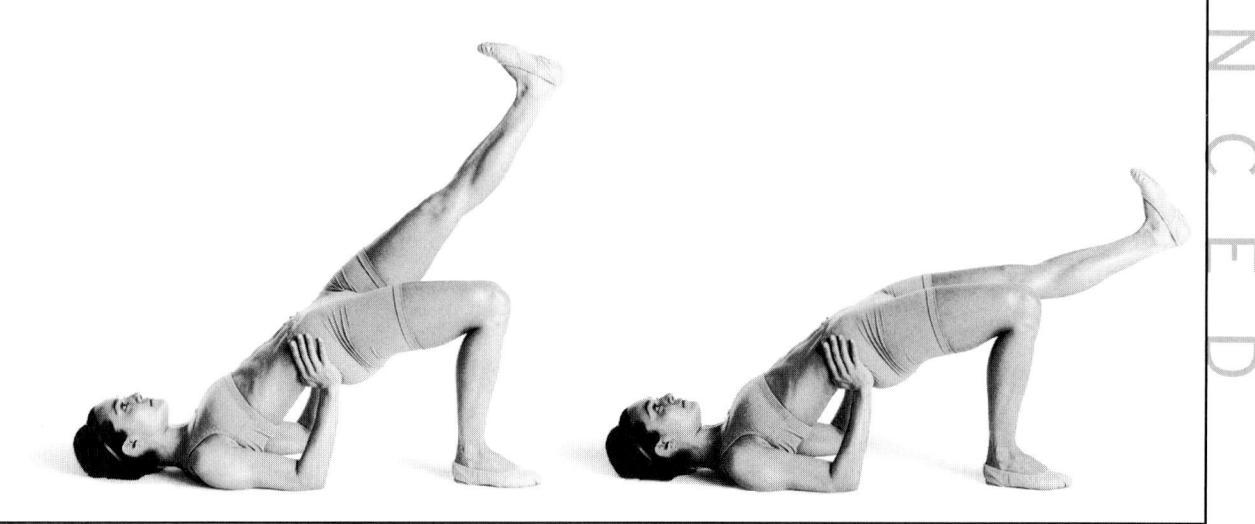

ADVANCED

SPINE TWIST

Step by Step

1. Sit up very tall with your arms stretched to either side of the room, and press the crown of your head up to the ceiling.
2. Straighten your legs out in front of you and glue them together in the Pilates stance with your feet flexed and your heels pressing out from under you.
3. Inhale and press your navel up and into your spine, as if you were being cinched at the waist.
4. Exhale and twist your torso to the right, staying perched on top of your hips and squeezing your buttocks and legs together tightly.
5. *Imagine you are a twisting vine growing taller from your roots.*
6. Increase the stretch by lifting up in the chest as you increase the exhalation.
7. Inhale deeply as you return to your starting position. Keep your shoulders pressing down and your arms outstretched.
8. Repeat the movement to the left and try to *imagine you are wringing the air out of your body as you would the water from a wet towel.*
9. Complete three sets and end by lying on your back with your arms by your sides to prepare for the Jackknife. . . .

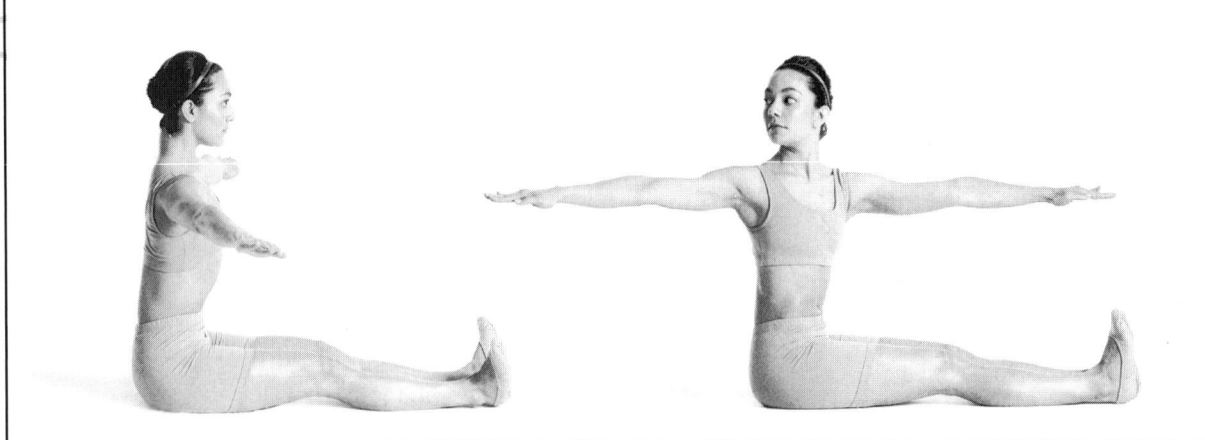

The Spine Twist is a breathing exercise used to wring the stale air from your lungs as you stretch the muscles of your back.

The Inside Scoop

GOAL
- To "wring" the stale air from your lungs as you twist without allowing your hips or heels to shift position.

KEYS
- Keep your feet flexing, and keep energy pressing out from your heels. Keep your legs straight throughout.
- Use your breath to increase the stretch, and focus as much on sitting tall in between the twists as while twisting.
- To ensure that you are twisting from your waist and not your shoulders, try placing your hands behind your head, one on top of the other, and repeating the movements. Remember to stay lifted in your chest.
- Squeeze your buttocks and upper inner thighs tightly together as you perform the sequence.
- Make sure to fill your lungs back up with new air as you return to center.
- Lengthen your neck and spine by pressing up from the crown of your head.

NO-NOS
- Do not sink into your back as you twist. Lift tall out of your waist and lift your chest as you go.
- Allow your head to follow the natural twist of the spine. Do not force your head to turn past the point of comfort.

VARIATION
- Add a slight pulse to each side to release the air from your lungs or sustain one long exhalation as you go.

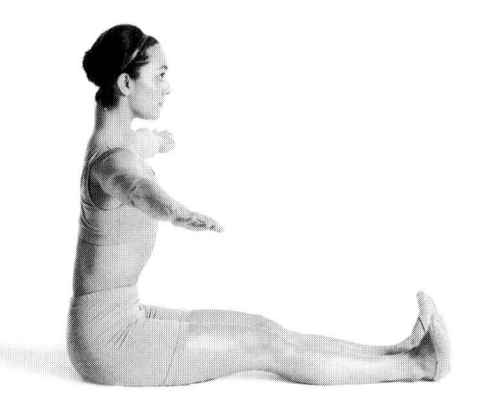

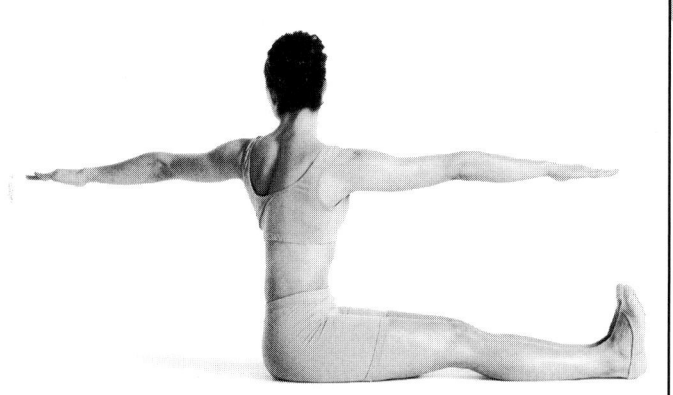

ADVANCED
THE JACKKNIFE

Step by Step

1. Lie on your back with your arms long and heavy by your sides and your legs straight out on the mat in the Pilates stance.
2. Inhale and press your navel deep down into your spine to initiate the movement of the Jackknife.
3. Squeezing your buttocks and the backs of the upper inner thighs together, lift your legs off the mat and bring them over your head by lifting from the back of the hips and engaging the powerhouse. Stop when you reach the back of your shoulders. Do not roll onto your neck.
4. From this position press the backs of your arms firmly into the mat, squeeze your buttocks tighter, and push your hips upward, raising your straight legs to the ceiling *as if opening a Swiss Army knife and snapping it into place*.
5. Keep your weight resting on the backs of your shoulders, and keep your feet in line with your nose.
6. Slowly begin rolling your spine back down to the mat vertebra by vertebra, exhaling as you go. Try to keep your hips and feet suspended in the air for as long as possible as you roll down, resisting gravity.
7. *Imagine your feet are supported by springs overhead.*
8. When your back is flat, stretch your legs toward the floor and then repeat the sequence. Inhale as you lift your legs and hips up, and exhale as you lower them back down to the mat.
9. Repeat three times and end by bringing your knees into your chest. Stretch yourself out and roll onto your side to prepare for the Side Kick Series. . . .

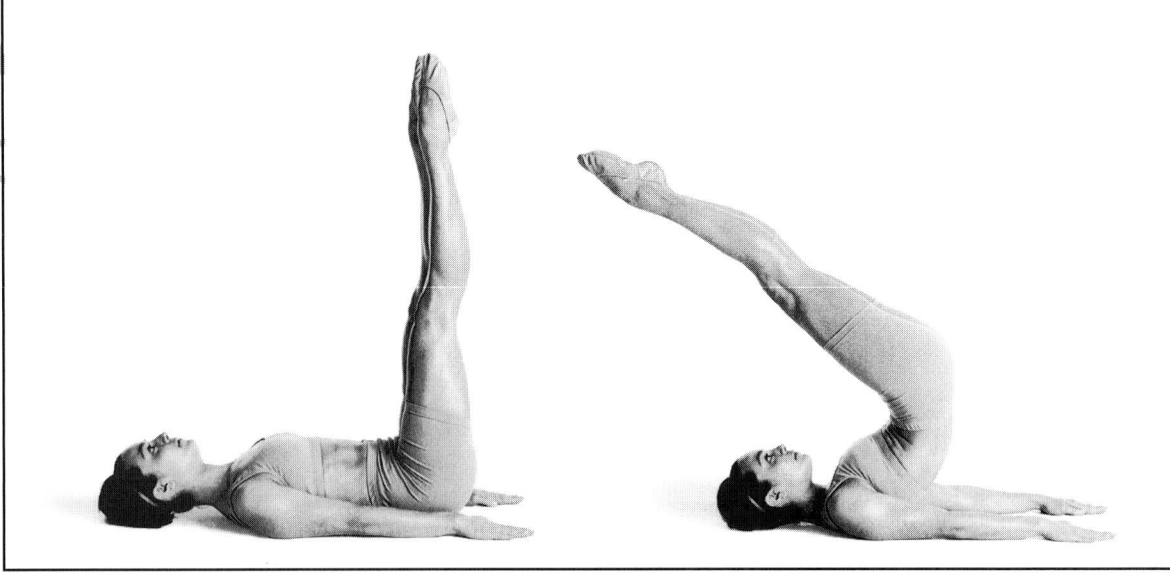

The Jackknife builds strength in your powerhouse and arms while stretching the muscles of your back, neck, and shoulders.

The Inside Scoop

If you have a bad neck, shoulder, or back, leave this exercise out.

GOAL
- To use the muscles of your powerhouse to keep your feet directly over your nose as you roll down.

KEYS
- Keep pressing your palms and the backs of your arms down into the mat as you lift your hips.
- Sliding your palms forward as you return your back down to the mat will help to stabilize your torso and release the muscles in your neck and shoulders.
- Pull your navel deep into your spine and use your exhalation to press deeper into the mat.
- Keep a slight turnout in your legs throughout the sequence to fully engage your hips and buttocks.

NO-NOS
- Do not roll onto your neck. Rest the weight of your body on the backs of your shoulders instead.
- Do not allow your legs to separate. Keep squeezing up the backs of the upper inner thighs and buttocks to support your lower back.

PROGRESSION
- As you progress you do not need to bring your legs all the way overhead before snapping up into your lifted position. Try to refine the angles of the movements to create a fluid motion of lifting and lowering.

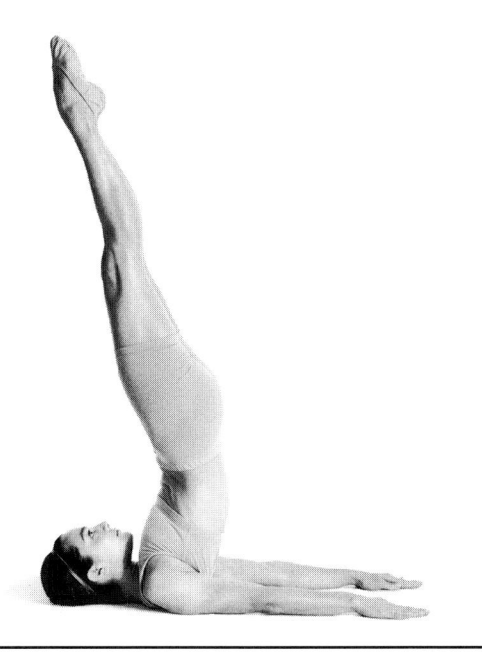

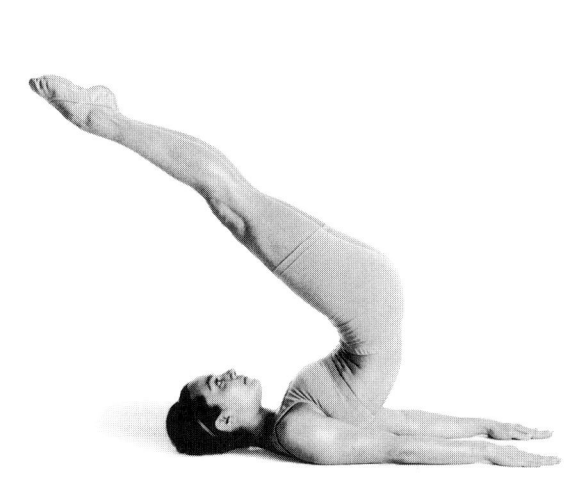

THE SIDE KICK SERIES

1. Front/Back
2. Up/Down
3. Small Circles
4. Side Passé
5. Inner-Thigh Lifts
6. Bicycle
7. Grande Ronde de Jambe
8. Transition: Heel Beats

The body position for the Side Kick Series remains the same throughout each exercise. With the exception of the inner-thigh lifts (p. 108) you should remain in one of the two upper-body positions shown at right. (If your neck or shoulder bothers you in these positions, see the modification.)

BODY POSITION
Step by Step

1. Lie on your side with your elbow, shoulder, midback, and buttocks aligned with the back edge of your mat.
2. Position your legs at a forty-five-degree angle in front of your body. (Adjust this position accordingly in the beginning until you feel you are able to maintain stability in this position. Think shoulder over shoulder, hip over hip.)
3. Keep your weight pressing into the palm of your forward hand and *imagine you are balancing a hot cup of coffee on your shoulder throughout the entire series*. (If you are in the advanced position, *imagine your top elbow is stuck to the ceiling*.)
4. Lengthen the back of your neck by pressing the crown of your head away from your shoulders.
5. Keep your feet in the Pilates stance with a *slight* turnout in the hip and thigh. (This will release your quadriceps and allow you to work from your hips and buttocks more efficiently.)
6. Your foot should be held long and aligned with your hip. (For variation, try pointing or flexing your foot to accentuate the movements. Remember, though, the exercises initiate from your hips and powerhouse, so do not focus too much on your lower leg.)

BODY POSITION
The Inside Scoop

The Side Kick Series works your inner and outer thighs and increases strength and mobility in the hip joint.

- The goal of this series is to gradually increase your range of motion, so do not attempt big movements at the expense of control. If you are rocking unsteadily just to achieve big kicks, you will sacrifice the integrity and efficiency of the movements.
- The most important part of the Side Kick Series is holding the upper-body position still as you perform the movements.
- Remember to use your powerhouse to stabilize your torso.
- In the beginning it is best to keep your forward hand pressing down into the mat in front of you (see beginner position below).
- Keep your weight pressing onto your bottom hip and make sure you are not rocking back and forth on your hip as you go.
- If your hip pops as you perform some of the movements, readjust your leg position and make sure you are squeezing your buttocks for control.
- Remember not to sink into your shoulders as you perform the series.
- If your neck gets tired or hurts during the series, simply lay your head down on your arm. (You can place a rolled-up towel or small pillow between your neck and your bottom arm to maintain the alignment of the spine in this position.)

Beginner

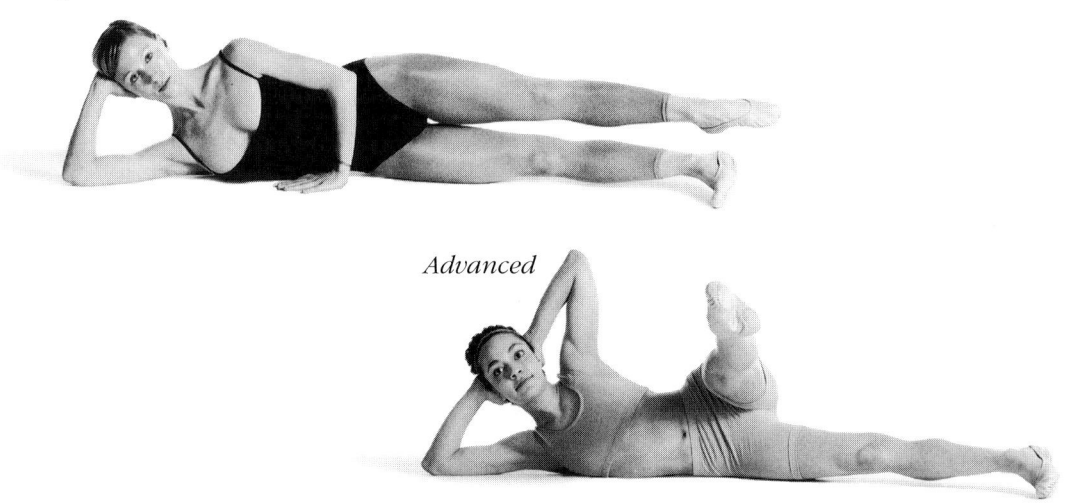

Advanced

INTERMEDIATE
FRONT/BACK

Step by Step

1. Take the Side Kick position (described on p. 98) that best suits your ability.
2. Lift your top leg to hip height and turn it out ever so slightly from the the hip to disengage the thigh.
3. Inhale, pressing your navel deep into your spine.
4. Swing your leg to the front and pulse it twice (like two small kicks) as far forward as it will go without rocking forward in your hips or scrunching in your waist.
5. Exhale as you swing your leg back, reaching for the back corner of the room.
6. *Imagine balancing cups of hot coffee on your shoulder and do not rattle the cups as you go.*
7. Repeat no more than ten times and bring your heels back together to prepare for Up/Down Kicks. . . .

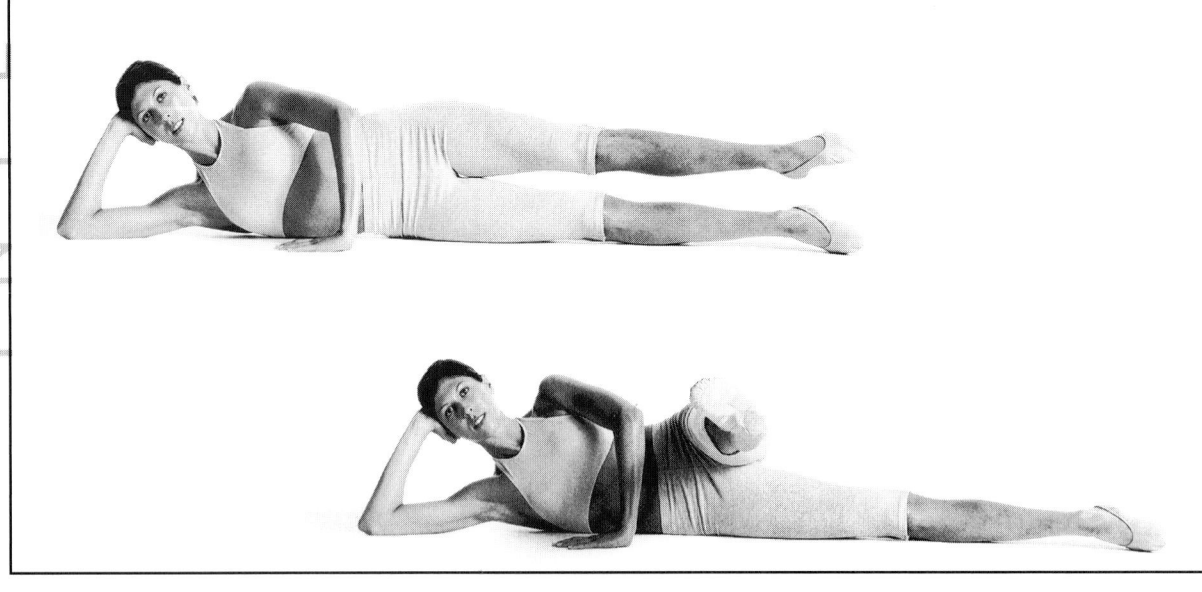

Front/Back Kicks work the back of your hips and buttocks, stretch your hamstrings, and improve balance.

The Inside Scoop

GOAL
- To maintain a long, perfectly stable torso as you swing your leg front and back.

KEYS
- Make sure your legs are long and straight without gripping your muscles.
- Use your powerhouse to stabilize your torso.

NO-NOS
- Do not allow your hips or shoulders to rock back and forth as you go.
- Do not allow your leg to bend completely or you will lose the stability in your hips.
- Do not let your foot or leg drop below the height of your hip as you perform the sequence.

PROGRESSION
- Begin with small kicks front and back and gradually increase your range of motion without wobbling.

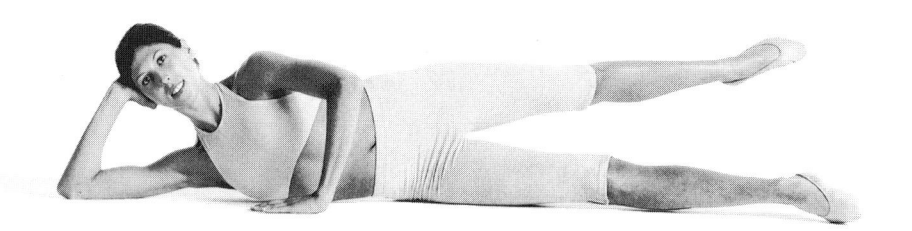

BEGINNER

UP/DOWN

Step by Step

1. Take the Side Kick position that best suits your ability. Keep your leg slightly turned out to disengage the quadriceps.
2. Inhale and lift your top leg straight up to the ceiling.
3. Exhale as you resist gravity on the way back down, stretching your leg long out of your hip as you go.
4. *Imagine your ankle is attached to a spring overhead* and use your powerhouse to control the movements.
5. Complete five sets and rest your heels together in the Pilates stance to prepare for the Small Circles. . . .

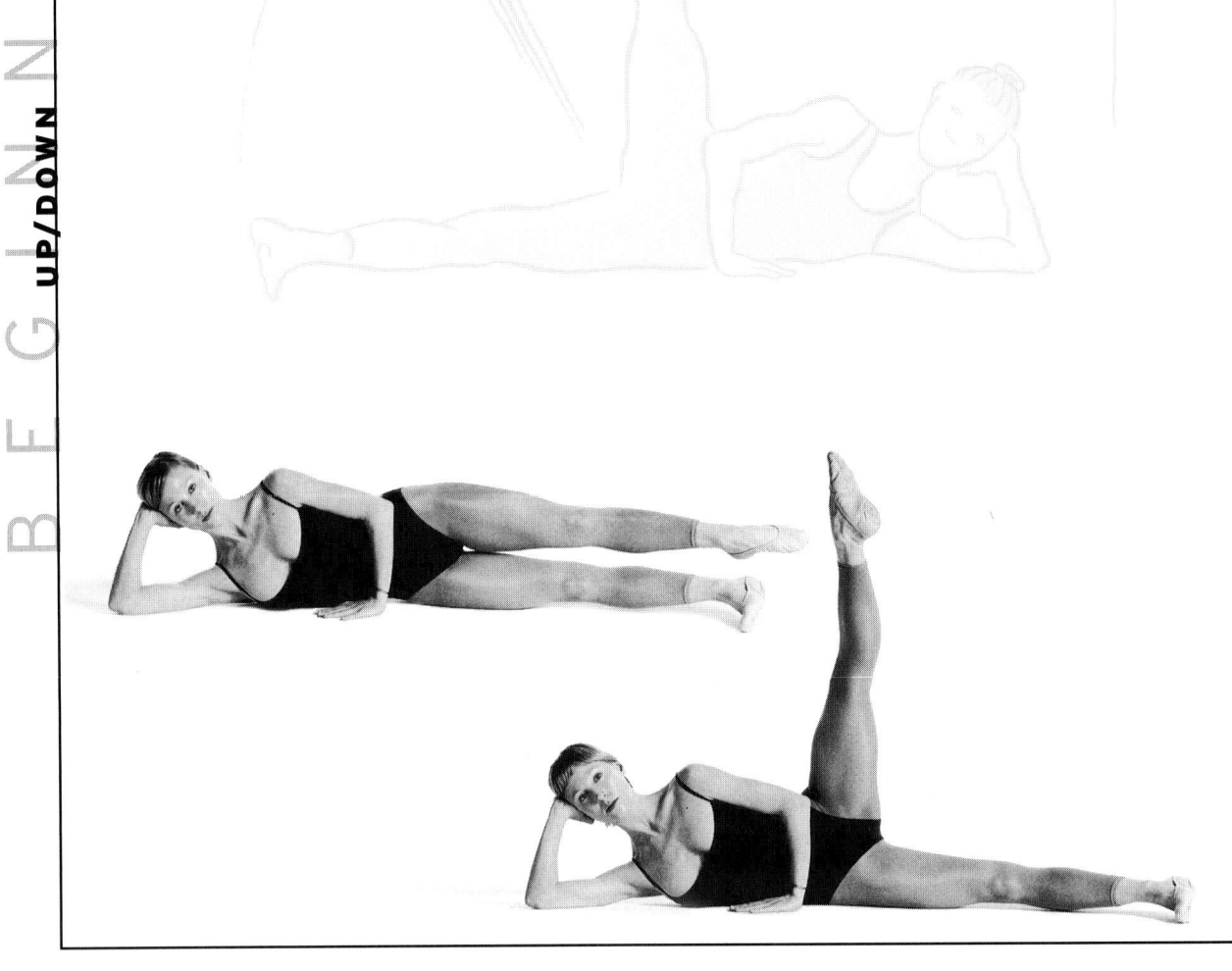

Up/Down Kicks work the hips, buttocks, and outer thighs and stretch your inner thigh muscles.

The Inside Scoop

- To remain long and lifted in your torso as you kick your leg up and lengthen it back down.
- Your leg will be tempted to roll inward during this movement, so be sure to keep a slight turnout in the hip and thigh throughout.
- Lift your leg only as high as you can manage with it remaining straight.
- Remember to lengthen your leg from the hip on the way back down, as if you are pressing away from your torso.
- *Imagine sliding a penny up the wall with your foot and pressing it into the wall on the way back down.*
- Stay lifted in your upper body by pressing the crown of your head away from your hips.
- Do not sink into your waist or shoulders as you lift your leg to the ceiling.

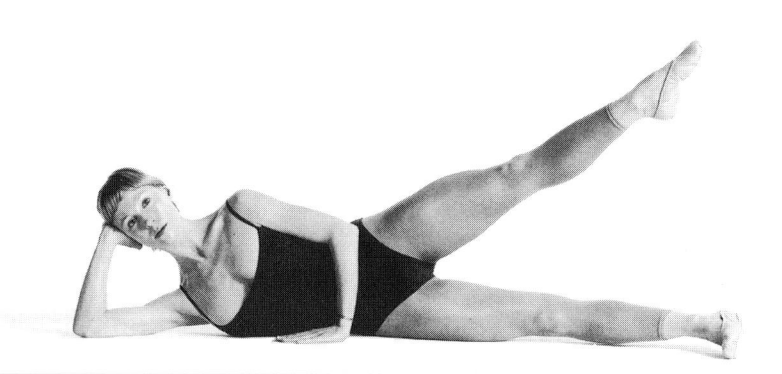

BEGINNER

SMALL CIRCLES

Step by Step

1. Take the Side Kick position that best suits your ability.
2. Lift your top heel just above your bottom heel and begin circling the leg from the hip in a small but vigorous forward motion.
3. *Imagine you are circling your leg inside a small hoop.*
4. Complete five circles forward and then reverse for five circles. End by resting the heels together in the Pilates stance.

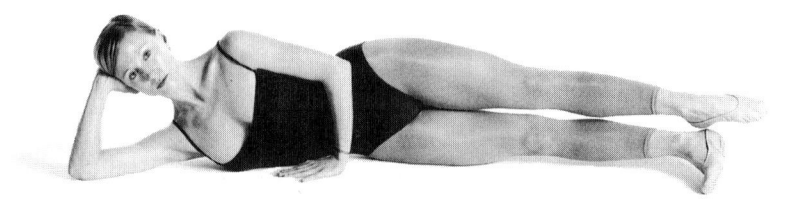

The Small Circles work the back of the hips, the buttocks, and the thighs.

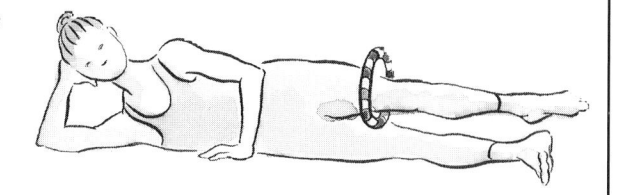

The Inside Scoop

GOAL
- To maintain perfectly still and lifted in your torso as you circle your leg.

KEYS
- Work the circles from the top of the leg and hip joint, keeping your leg straight as you do so.
- Lengthen your leg from the hip *as if pressing a penny into the wall with your foot.*
- Squeeze your buttocks for support.
- Use your powerhouse to maintain stability in your torso so you do not rock back and forth.

NO-NOS
- Do not allow your knee, thigh, or foot to roll inward as you go.
- Do not bend your knee or circle from your lower leg; work from the hip down.

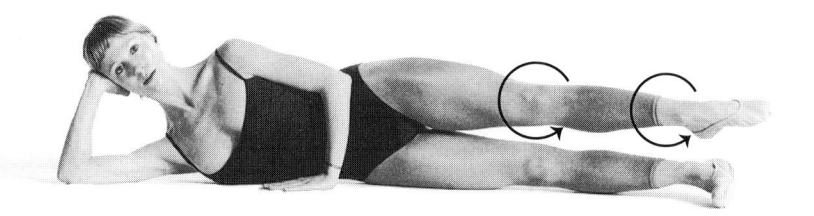

INTERMEDIATE
SIDE PASSÉ

Step by Step

1. Take the Side Kick position that best suits your ability.
2. Lift your top leg straight up to the ceiling. Bend your knee and bring your foot down to the inside of the opposite thigh or just in front of it. Slide your foot down the length of the leg until it is straight, and then lift it up to the ceiling again. Maintain a long leg and foot.
3. Repeat three to five times and then reverse the motion, drawing the foot into the body, lifting it straight to the ceiling, and then resisting gravity as you lower it down to the stationary leg.
4. *Imagine your leg resisting the pull of a spring attached overhead.*
5. Repeat three to five times in each direction. On the last repetition draw the foot in toward the body and place it on the floor just in front of your bottom thigh to prepare for the Inner-Thigh Lifts. . . .

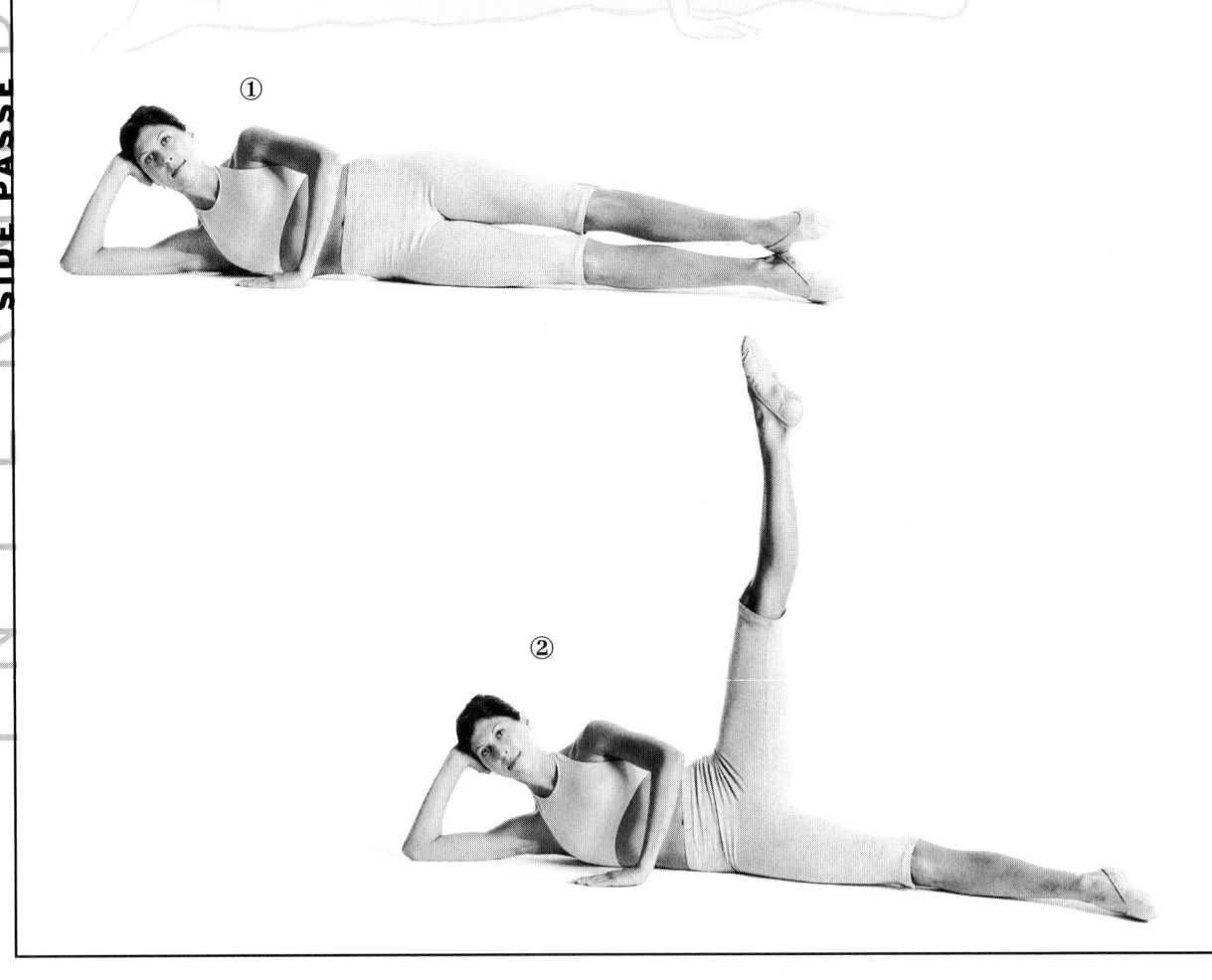

This exercise is adapted from the spring work usually performed on the apparatus. It works the hips and inner and outer thighs.

The Inside Scoop

- To maintain a long and perfectly stable torso as you perform the sequence.

- Rhythm! Allow the fluidity and feeling of the movements to enrich the exercise.
- The more still you remain in your torso, the more efficient the exercise will be.
- Stay lengthened in your waistline throughout.
- Reach your leg long out of your hip *as if you were pressing a penny into the wall with your foot.*

- Do not sink into your shoulder or waist as you straighten your leg to the ceiling.
- Do not allow your knee, thigh, or foot to roll inward as you go.

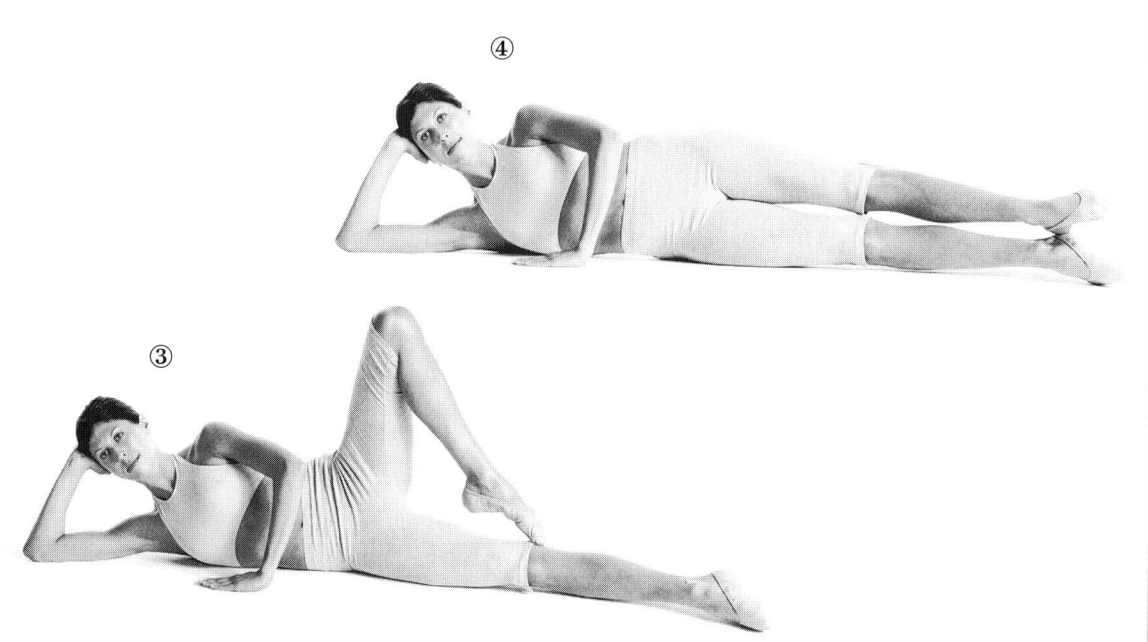

INTERMEDIATE
INNER-THIGH LIFTS

Step by Step

1. Lie on your right side with your left foot crossed in front of your right leg, foot flat on the floor, and kneecap facing the ceiling.
2. Rest your head on your arm and with the other hand take hold of your ankle to hold it in place, or press your palm down into the mat in front of you.
3. Extend your straight leg long out of your hip and raise it off the floor, turning your heel slightly toward the ceiling.
4. *Imagine you have a stack of books balanced on the inside of your knee as you go.*
5. Lift and lower your leg without letting it touch the mat. Emphasis is on the lifting.
6. Lower and lift five to ten times and then hold the leg in the lifted position, pulsing it upward for ten small pulses. *Do not drop the books!* You can also try five circles forward and five circles back in this lifted position. End by sliding your bent leg down the other and into the Pilates stance to prepare for the Bicycle. . . .

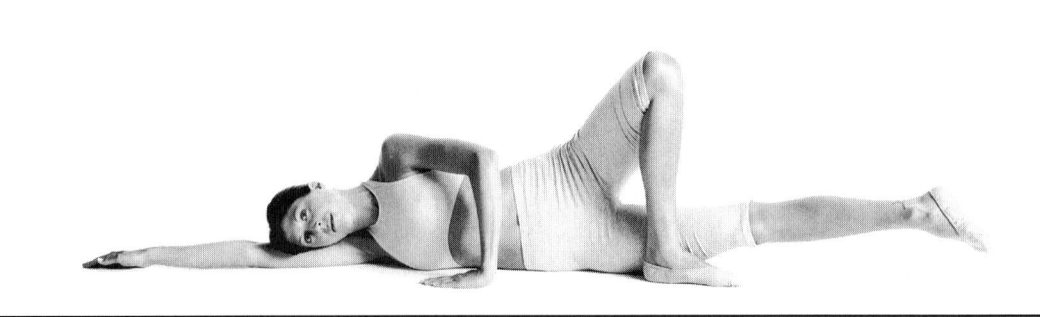

The Inner-Thigh Lifts work your inner and outer thighs and stretch the back of the hip.

The Inside Scoop

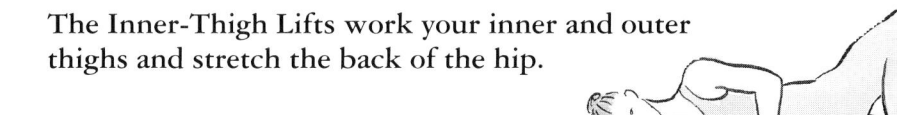

- To maintain an actively outstretched body as you perform the lifting movements.
- If it is too difficult to keep your upright leg bent in this position, simply rest your knee on the mat in front of you.
- Lift as much of your thigh off the mat as you can, maintaining a slight outward rotation of the leg.
- Maintain your long, steady upper body by stretching your outreached arm in opposition to your leg.
- Do not bend your outstretched leg as you go.
- Do not grip in your quadriceps.

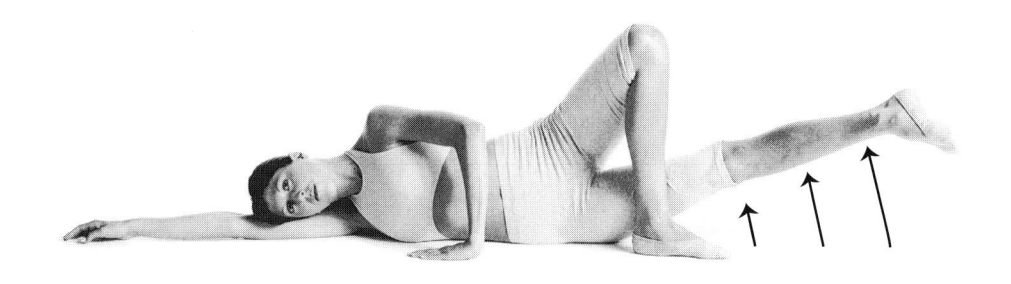

ADVANCED

BICYCLE

Step by Step

1. Take the Advanced Side Kick position.
2. Swing your top leg back *as if pushing on the pedal of a very large bicycle,* bending your knee behind you and bringing your heel to your buttock for a stretch in the hip and knee. Bring your bent knee past your outstretched knee and toward your shoulder, not dropping forward in your hips. Extend your leg out in front of you *as if pushing forward on the pedal* and "cycle" by swinging your straight leg back to repeat the motion.
3. *Try to envision the bicycle as being very large and hard to pedal so that you can control the movement and get the most from the stretch.*
4. Pedal forward three times and then reverse the sequence, pedaling backward three times. End by bringing your heels back together into the Pilates stance to prepare for the Grande Ronde de Jambe. . . .

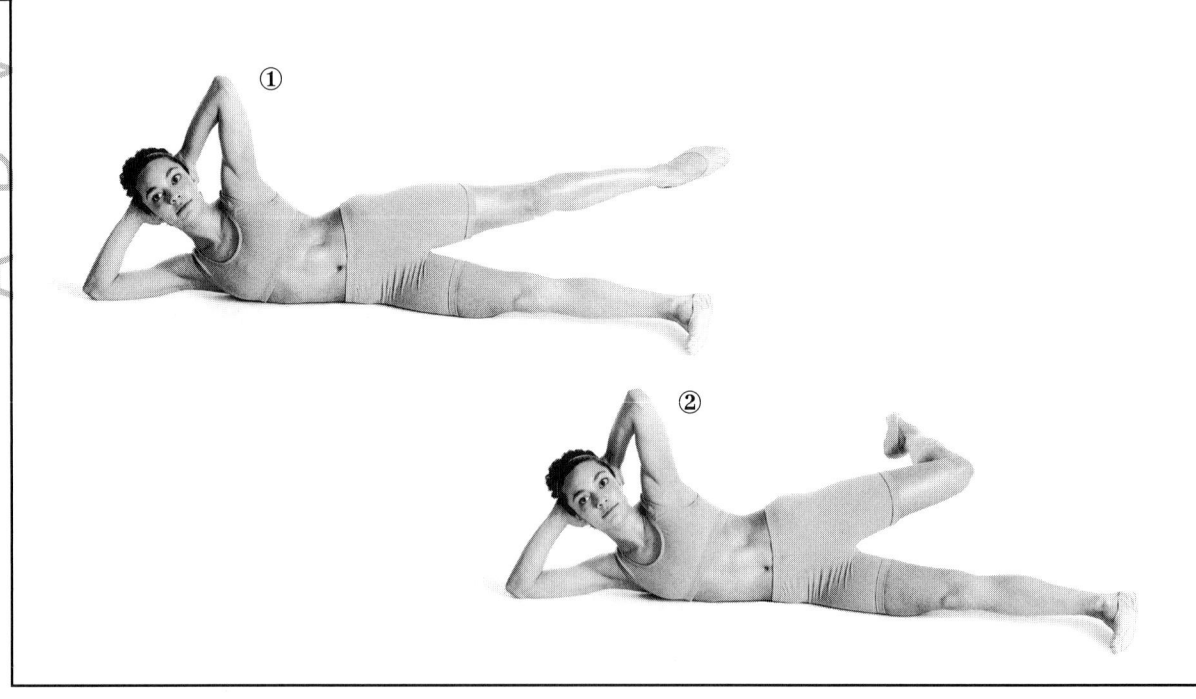

The Bicycle stretches and strengthens the hips, buttocks, and hamstrings.

The Inside Scoop

GOAL
- To maintain a long, perfectly stable torso as you cycle forward and back.

KEYS
- Stay long in your waistline throughout the movements, especially when holding your leg straight out in front of you.

   Cycling Backward (kick forward, bend knee, knee back, straighten leg)
- Press your knee as far back as possible before straightening your leg behind you.
- Lengthen your back as you stretch your leg.

   Cycling Forward (leg back, bend knee, knee forward, straighten leg)
- Bring your heel to your buttock *before* bringing your knee forward.

NO-NOS
- Do not allow your knee, thigh, or foot to roll inward as you stretch.
- Do not bring your hip forward as your leg swings to the front.
- Do not drop your leg below hip level.

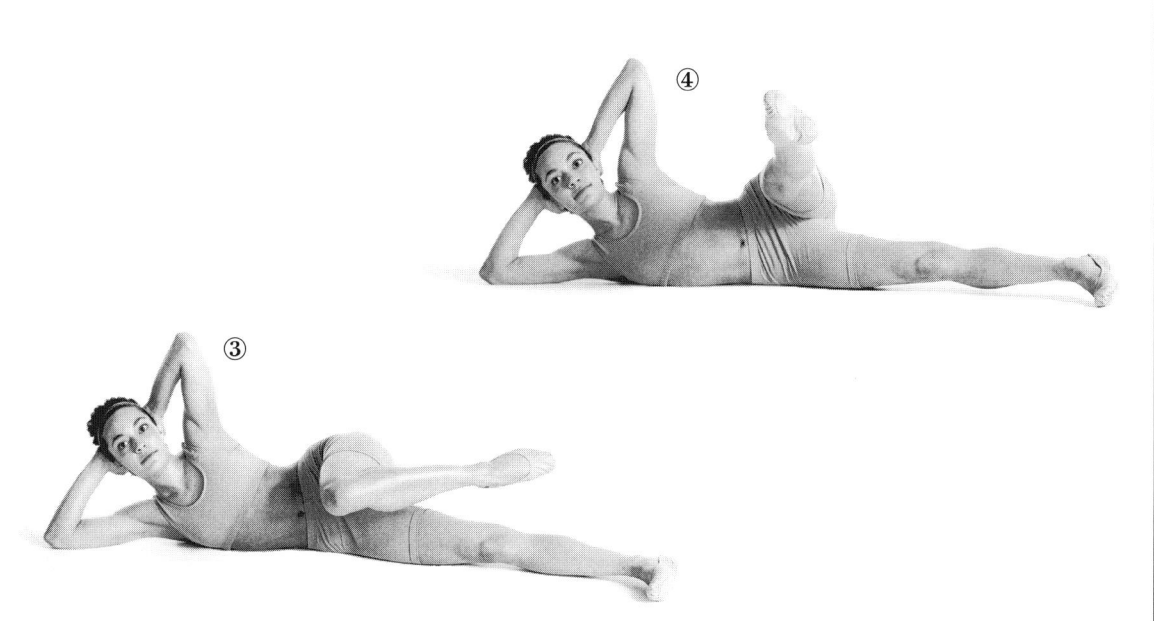

ADVANCED

BICYCLE

ADVANCED
GRANDE RONDE DE JAMBE

Step by Step

1. Take the Advanced Side Kick position.
2. Lift your top leg to hip height, keeping it slightly turned out.
3. Inhale and swing your leg to the front. Slide your foot up the wall in front of you, rotate the leg in your hip socket and reach back to the corner of the wall behind you. (Remember to press your top hip forward and stretch your upper back longer to create a counterbalance for the weight of the leg stretching back.)
4. Swing your leg to the front and repeat the sequence two or three times: swing forward, lift, rotate, and stretch back. *Imagine stirring the inside of a large cauldron.*
5. Reverse the sequence by swinging your leg back and long out of your hip. Lift your foot to the ceiling, rotating your leg outward in the hip socket. Lower your leg and hold it at hip height before repeating the sequence. Swing back, lift, rotate, and slowly lower to hip height. Remember to maintain a long, strong torso for stability as you perform these movements.
6. Repeat two or three times in each direction and end by bringing your heels together in the Pilates stance and rolling onto your stomach to prepare for Transition: Heel Beats. . . .

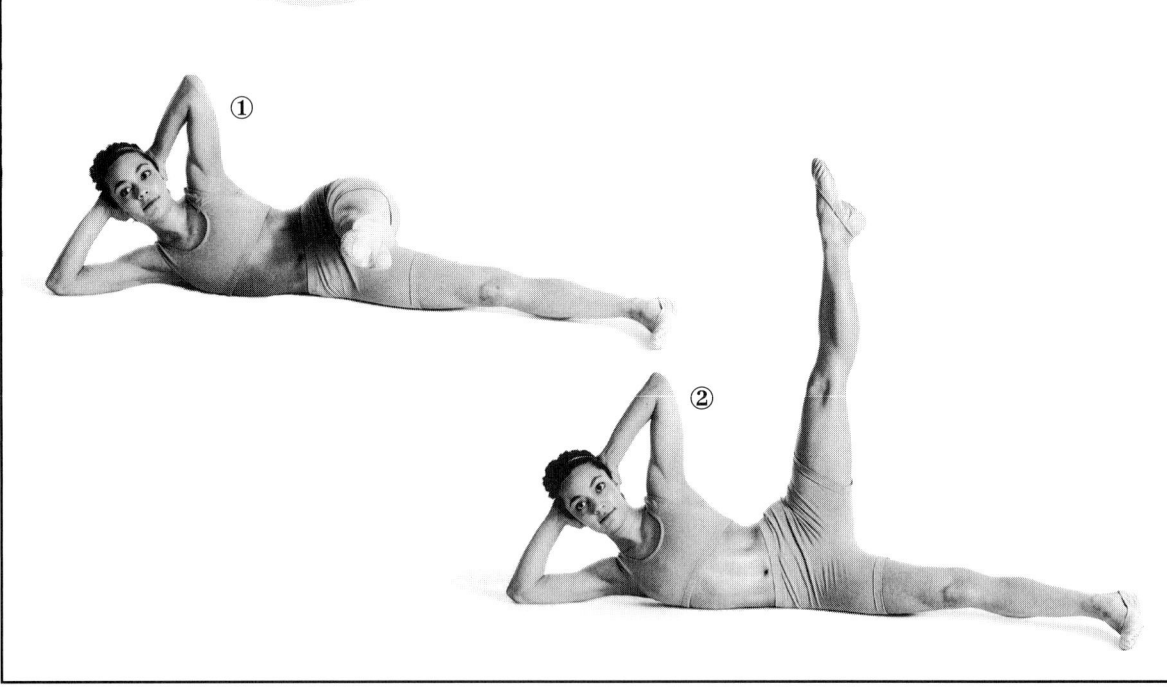

The Grande Ronde de Jambe articulates the leg within the hip joint, stretches the hamstrings and hip flexors, and works the powerhouse.

The Inside Scoop

- To maintain a long, stable torso as you circle your leg.
- Remember to counterbalance the weight of your leg by pressing your top hip in opposition to your foot.
- Keep energy pressing out the crown of your head, and keep pressing your shoulders down away from your ears.
- Do not sink into your waist or shoulders as you go.
- Do not allow yourself to rock in the hips.

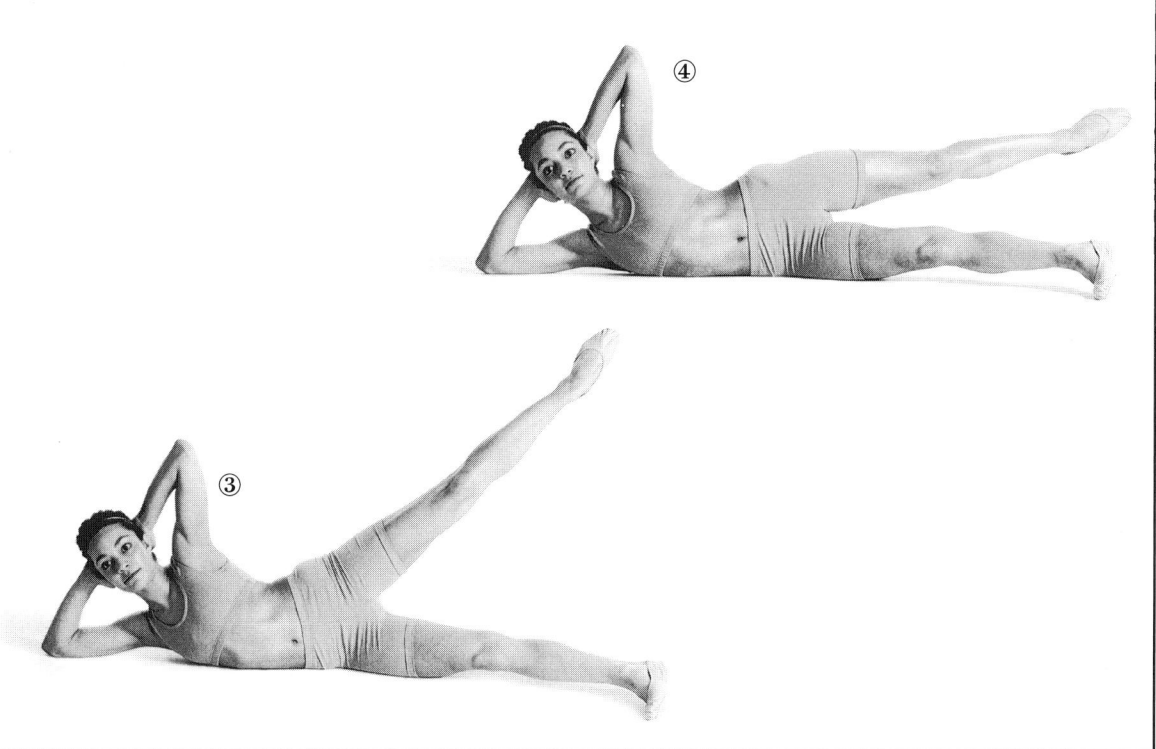

INTERMEDIATE
Transition: HEEL BEATS

Step by Step

1. Lie on your stomach, squeezing the backs of your legs together, and rest your forehead on the back of your hands (one on top of the other).
2. Squeeze your buttocks tight, inhale, and lift both thighs off the mat behind you, keeping your legs straight and heels together.
3. Hold your legs in the air and beat your heels together lightly.
4. *Imagine your upper body is strapped to the mat, unable to move, and your legs are suspended by springs behind you.*
5. Inhale for five beats and exhale for five beats.
6. End by sitting back onto your heels to release your lower back, and then lie on your other side in the Side Kick position.

   NOTE: For an advanced variation, try bringing your heels into your buttocks and then straightening your legs with your thighs still lifted. Repeat three times. (See variation photo.)

7. Repeat the Side Kick Series exercises with the opposite leg and end by lying on your back with your knees pulled into your chest to prepare for the Teasers. . . .

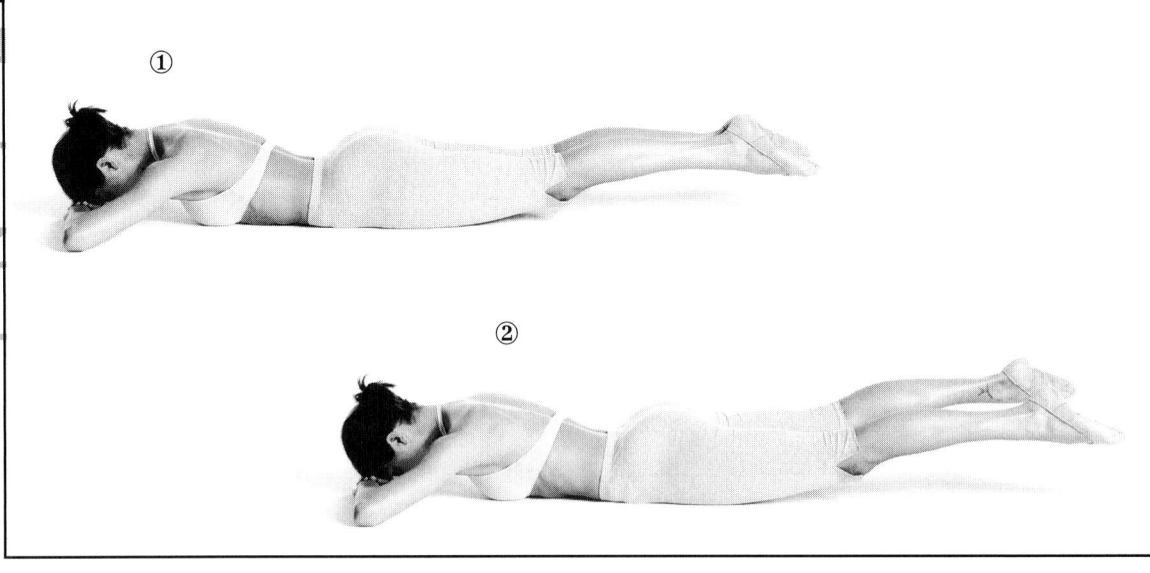

The Heel Beats work your powerhouse and the backs of your legs.

The Inside Scoop

- To remain perfectly still in your torso with your legs raised and beating, or bending and straightening.

- Keep your navel pulled up into your spine to protect your lower back.
- Keep your upper back and shoulders relaxed during the beats. If you need to, reach your arms out long in front of you.
- Squeeze your buttocks tight to protect your lower back and stabilize your torso.
- Keep your legs as straight as possible throughout the beats.
- Keep your knees as lifted as possible throughout the Advanced Variation.

- Do not beat your heels so vigorously as to bruise them. Work from the whole leg.
- Make sure your thighs are not touching the mat as you go.

Advanced Variation

①

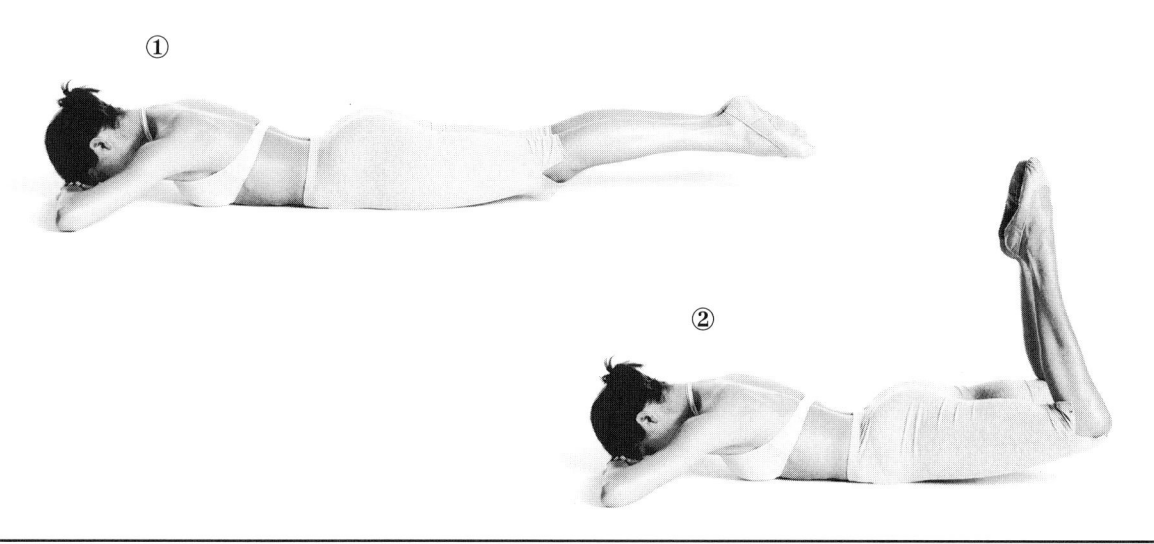

②

TEASER (Preparation I)

Step by Step

1. Lie on your back and place the soles of your feet flat on the mat with your knees and thighs squeezing together. (Your feet should be at a forty-five-degree angle from your knees.)
2. Reach your arms back overhead and stretch your fingertips to the back wall. Maintain a flat back by engaging your powerhouse.
3. Bring your arms forward and allow your head and upper body to begin following them forward and up. *Imagine you are being lifted by a balloon attached to your chest.*
4. Inhaling, roll up to where your abdominals are still engaged and hold yourself there for a count of three.
5. As you exhale, begin rolling your spine back down, pressing each vertebra into the mat as you go.
6. When the back of your head has touched down, begin reaching your arms back over your head and stretch your fingertips to the wall behind you. Maintain a long neck as you do so.
7. Repeat this sequence three times and then go on to Teaser Preparation II. . . .

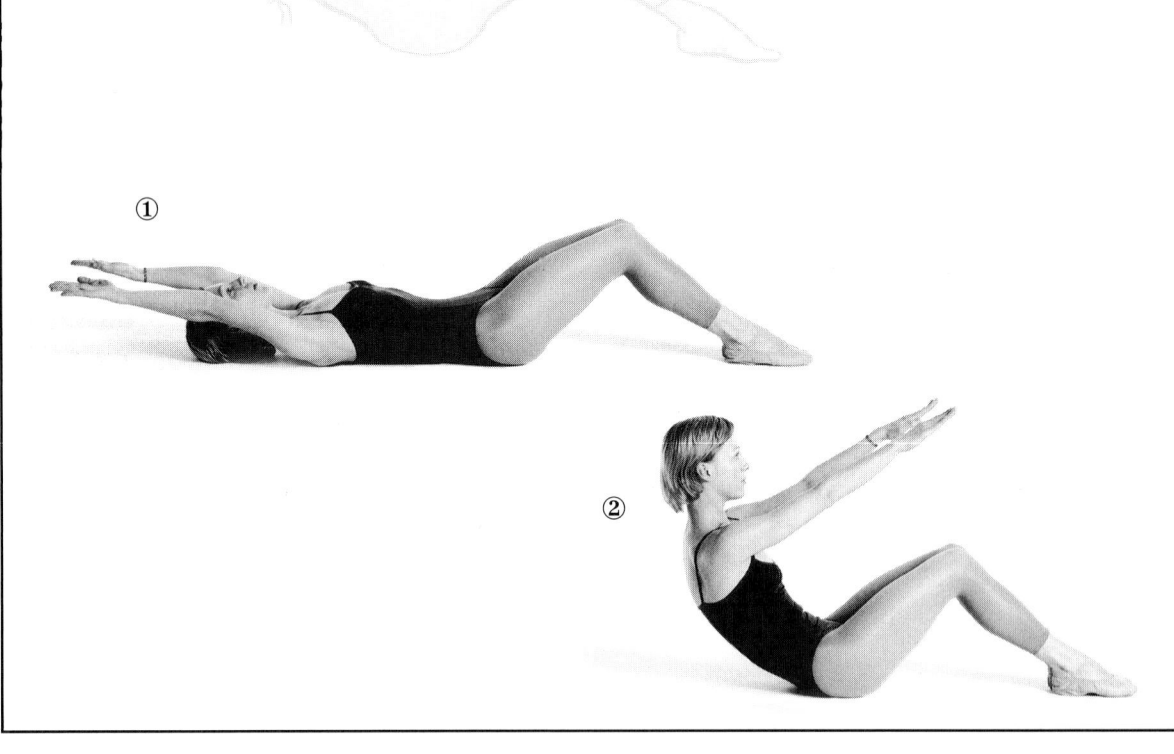

This variation is meant to test the strength of your powerhouse before moving on to the full Teasers.

The Inside Scoop

- To remain perfectly still in your lower body while rolling up and lowering yourself back down.

- Try to focus on lifting up more than forward to keep your powerhouse engaged.
- Keep squeezing your buttocks, inner thighs, and knees together throughout.
- Lengthen as you roll down, keeping your sacrum pressed flat to the mat.

- Do not allow your feet to move as you roll up.
- Do not rock forward onto your tailbone.

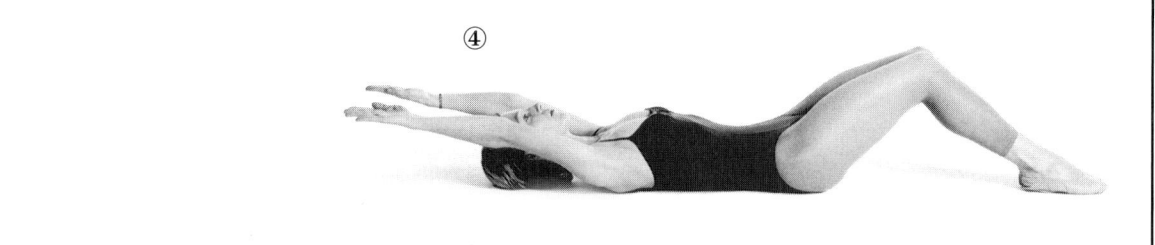

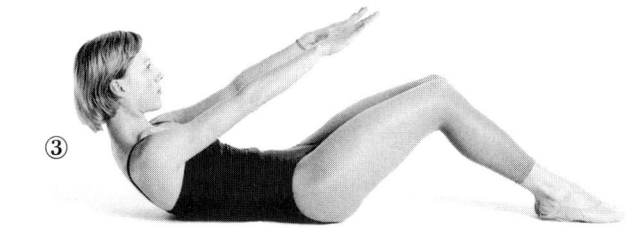

TEASER (Preparation II)

Step by Step

1. Lie on your back, remaining in the position of the Teaser (Preparation I).
2. Straighten one leg up to a forty-five-degree angle from the floor and glue it to the inside of your opposite knee. Turn out slightly in the hip and thigh and squeeze your buttocks and inner thighs together tightly.
3. Repeat the same sequence as in Preparation I without allowing your knees to come apart as you go.
4. Reach for your outstretched foot, staying lifted in your chest. Lift tall out of your waist as you inhale. *Imagine being pulled up by the force of a magnet.*
5. As you exhale, begin rolling your spine down to the mat and stretch your arms back overhead.

   NOTE: For an abdominal challenge, when you reach the top, exhale and twist your upper body to the right. Inhale and return to center, then exhale and twist to the left. Inhale and return to center. Exhaling, lower yourself slowly back down to the mat.

6. Repeat either variation two or three times with each leg and end by pulling your knees into your chest and releasing your back before going on to the full Teasers. . . .

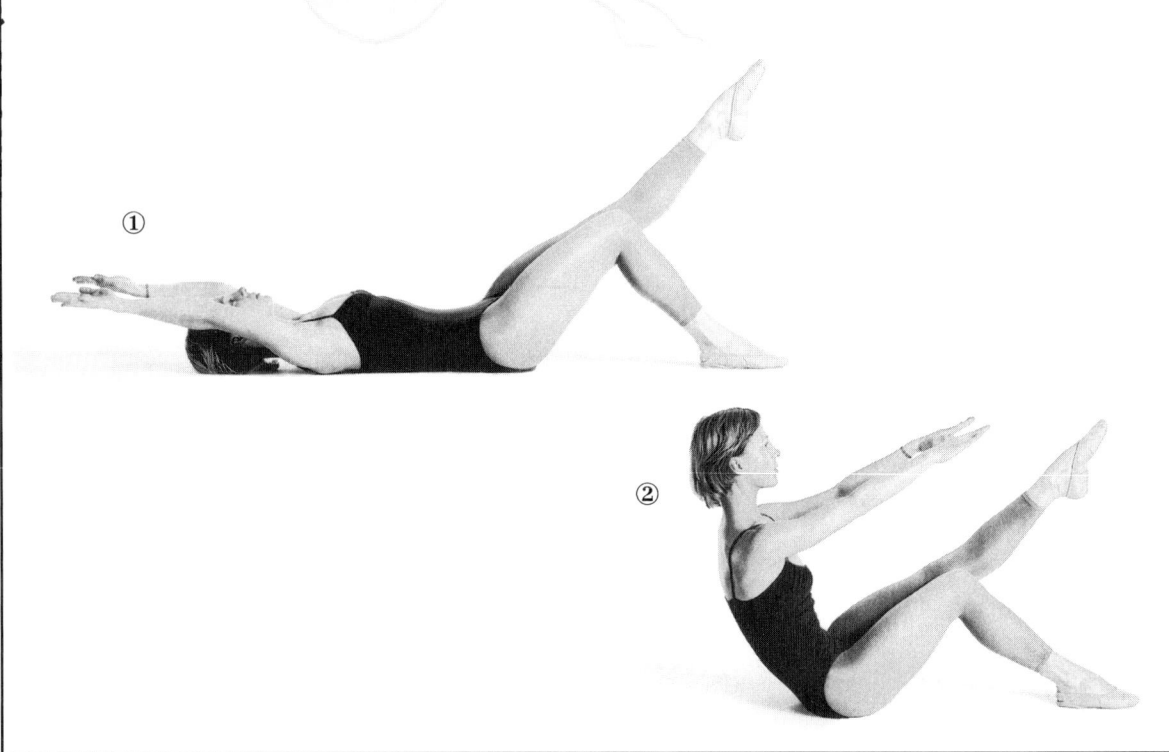

This variation works your powerhouse and stabilizes your lower body in preparation for the full Teaser.

The Inside Scoop

GOAL

- To keep your knees glued together and your leg straight throughout the sequence.

KEYS

- Work from the deep muscles of your powerhouse to control the movement.
- The key to getting up to the top is to feel yourself "floating" slowly upward with control.
- Think of lifting from your chest and pressing your shoulders down and away from your ears.
- Remember to articulate your spine as you roll up and down, creating space between each vertebra.

NO-NOS

- Make sure your knees do not come unglued as you perform these movements. (And no cheating by resting one knee on top of the other!)
- Do not allow your shoulders to creep up around your ears as you lift upward. Do not hold your breath or throw your body weight upward.

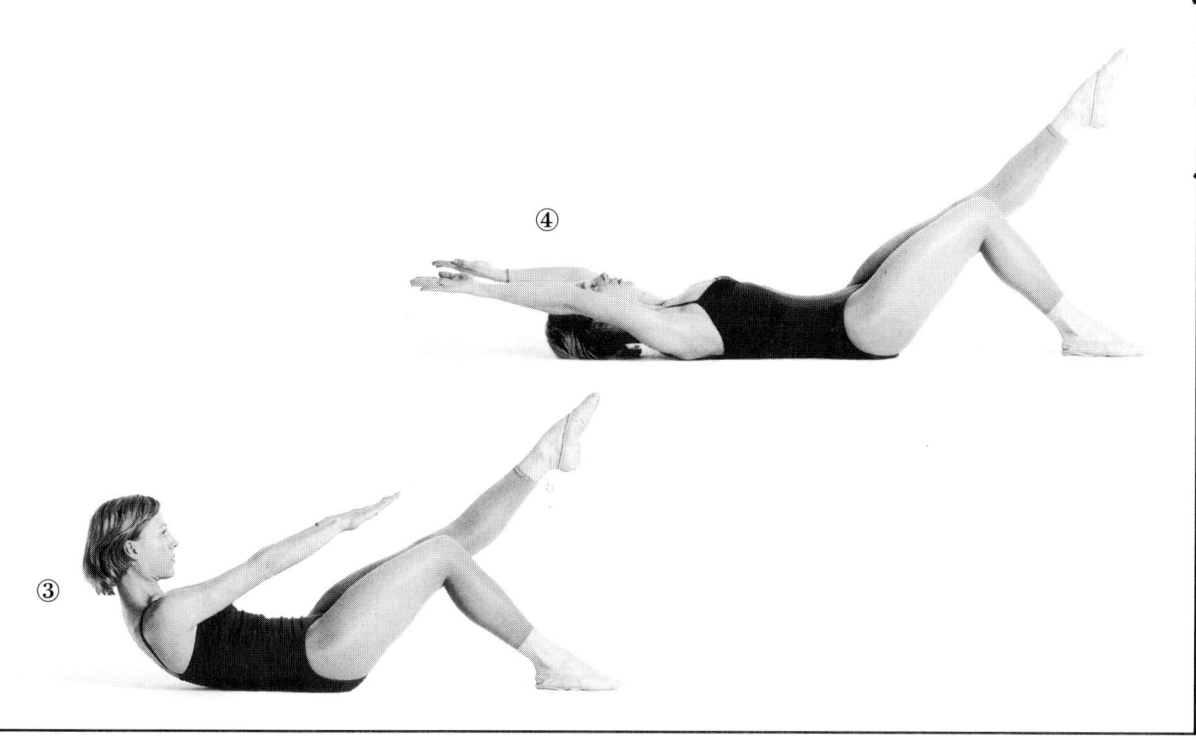

TEASER (Preparation II)

INTERMEDIATE
TEASER I

Step by Step

1. Lie on your back with both legs straight to the ceiling and in the Pilates stance.
2. Stretch your arms long overhead while maintaining a flat back.
3. Lower your legs to a forty-five-degree angle from the floor, pressing your navel deeper into your spine.
4. Inhale and bring your arms from over your head to reach toward your toes.
5. Allow your body to "float" up to your feet by bringing your chin to your chest and "peeling" your upper body off the mat.
6. *Imagine you have a spring attached from your ankles to your chest that pulls you up toward your feet.*
7. Hold that V position, balancing on your tailbone, and then exhale as you begin rolling your spine back down to the mat. *Feel the pull of the spring as you descend in opposition.* Squeeze your buttocks tightly to make sure that your legs remain stationary.
8. When your head has touched down on the mat, stretch your arms out long overhead and repeat the sequence, inhaling as you float up and exhaling as you press each vertebra back into the mat beneath you.
9. Repeat the sequence three times and end by sitting up and placing the soles of your feet on the mat to prepare for the Seal. . . . (p. 140)

   NOTE: For the advanced level, end in the lifted V position to prepare for Teaser II. . . .

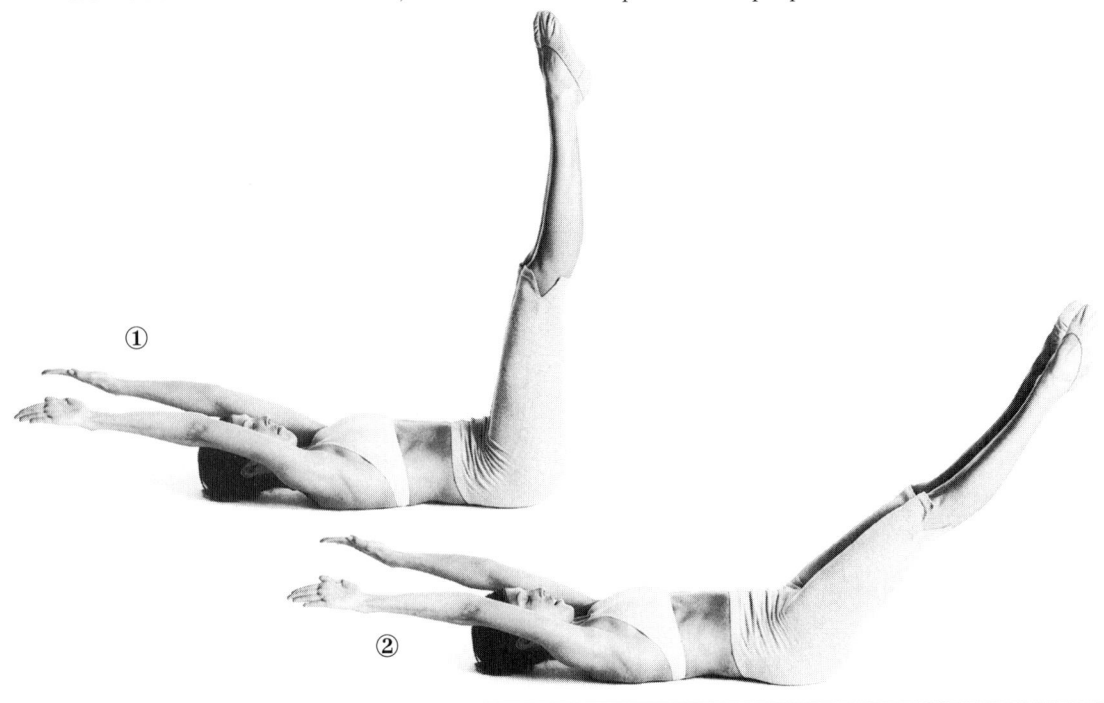

The Teaser I is one of the all-time favorites of the Pilates method. It tests your powerhouse control to the fullest and is a great way to chart your progress.

The Inside Scoop

If your back hurts, stop. Lie back with your knees into your chest to release your lower back.

- To remain perfectly still in your lower body as you perform the movements of the Teaser.

- The key to the Teaser series is to relax your mind and find your rhythm as you go.
- You must *breathe* during this sequence. If you hold your breath, you will not be using your muscles efficiently.
- Make sure to press your navel down deep into your spine and squeeze your buttocks and backs of the inner thighs to engage your powerhouse.

- Do not lower your legs past the point of control. If you feel your back beginning to arch off the mat, raise your legs back up toward the ceiling.
- The Teasers consist of very controlled movements. Do not allow yourself to "throw" your body up or drop it back down.

- Hold your arms straight to the ceiling, alongside your ears, as you roll down. Try to stretch away from your legs as you go.

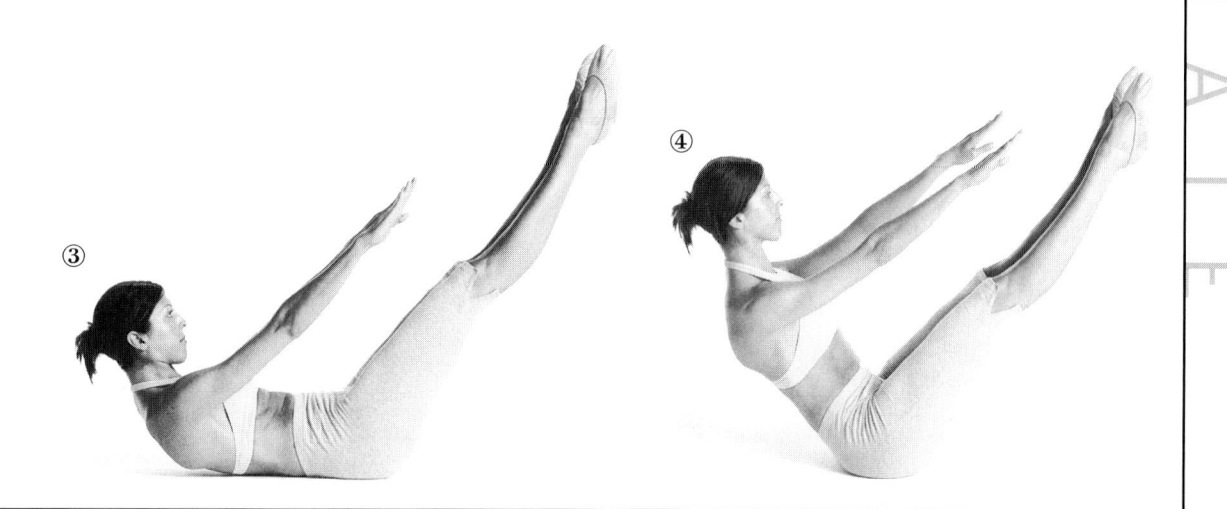

ADVANCED

TEASER II

Step by Step

1. You are in the lifted V position of Teaser I, balancing on your tailbone and pressing your navel deep into your spine.
2. Hold your upper body absolutely still as you lower your legs toward the mat.
3. Lower and lift your legs three times, making sure you are working from your powerhouse by keeping your navel pressed to your spine and squeezing your buttocks and inner thighs together tightly.
4. *Imagine your legs are pointed arrows hinged at your hips or suspended by springs, attached to your ankles, and are supported as you pull down on the springs and resist their pull on the way up.*
5. Inhale as you lower your legs and exhale as you return to your V position.
6. End in the lifted V position to prepare for Teaser III. . . .

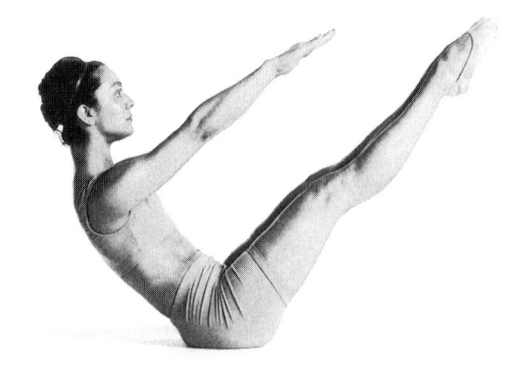

The Teaser II improves balance and coordination and works the powerhouse.

The Inside Scoop

If your back hurts, stop. Lie down and pull your knees to your chest to release your lower back.

- To maintain a rigid, lifted upper body as you lower and lift your legs with control.
- Make sure you are slightly turned out at the hip and thigh, Pilates stance, to engage the muscles of the inner thighs, hips, and buttocks.
- Keep lifted in your chest as if you were suspended from the ceiling. Think of lifting your legs to your chest as you bring them up each time.
- Press your shoulders down and away from your ears to release the neck and shoulder muscles.
- Total control is key, so make your movements slow and deliberate until you have it mastered.

- Do not allow yourself to rock forward and back on your tailbone.
- Do not allow your back to arch or sink as you lower your legs. Keep squeezing the backs of your legs and do not lower them past the point of control.
- Do not drop your legs.

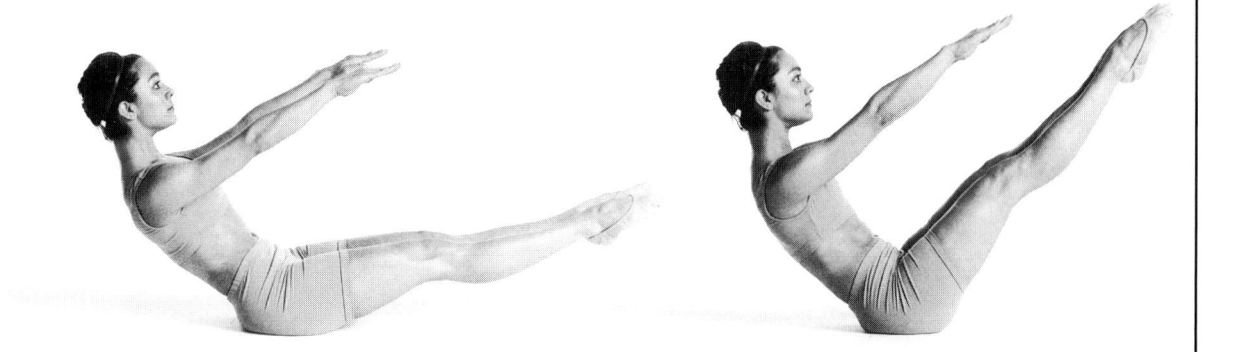

ADVANCED

TEASER III

Step by Step

1. You are in the lifted V position of Teaser II, balancing on your tailbone and pressing your navel deep into your spine.
2. Lift your arms to the ceiling alongside your ears and slowly roll your entire body back down to the mat. Initiate the roll down by pressing your navel deep into your spine and stretch in opposition as you go, reaching your upper back away from your ankles and allowing every vertebra to press down in between. Stretch your fingertips to the wall behind you.
3. Use the combined movements of Teasers I and II to begin folding back up into your V position, lifting the upper body and ankles off the mat simultaneously until your fingers touch your toes.
4. *Imagine resisting the pull of a heavy spring that is attached between your breastbone and your ankles or that you are two distinct arrows hinged at your hips.*
5. Stretch your arms up and back alongside your ears and exhale as you slowly begin stretching the spring back out, reaching your upper back away from your ankles, until you have pressed each vertebra back down into the mat beneath you.
6. Initiate the roll back down by pressing your navel deeper into your spine and squeezing up the back of the inner thighs and buttocks to support your lower back.
7. Repeat three times and end by holding yourself in the lifted V position. Bring your arms behind you and place them, palms down and fingers facing away from you, onto the mat to prepare for Hip Circles. . . .

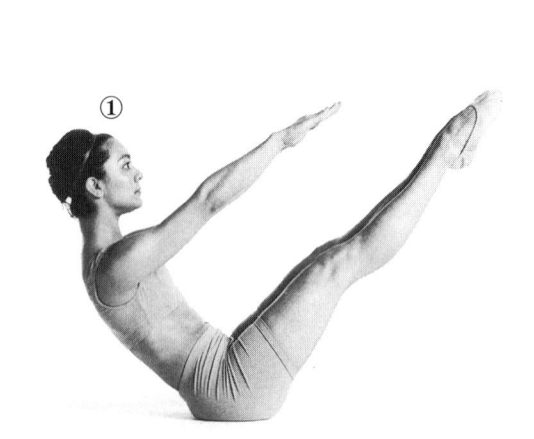

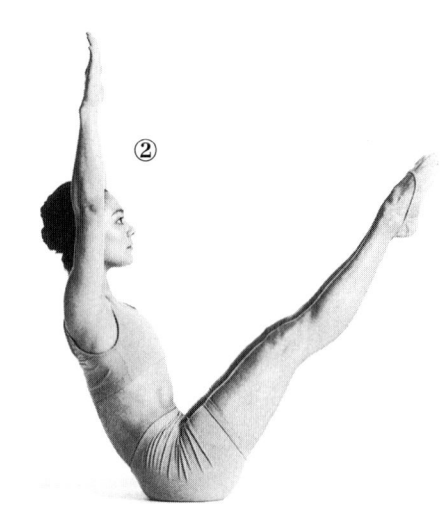

The Teaser III is the combination of Teasers I and II and utilizes all the muscles of the body with an accent on the powerhouse.

The Inside Scoop

If your back hurts, stop. Lie down and pull your knees into your chest to release your lower back.

- To stretch as long as possible and fold up as fully as possible using the control of your powerhouse.
- Make sure that you initiate the movement of Teaser III from your powerhouse.
- Think of folding up around your center by pressing your navel firmly to your spine and squeezing your buttocks to begin.
- Use the sensation of "floating" as you lift your body up into the V position.
- If you have trouble coming up, try reversing the breathing sequence.
- Keep your shoulders pressing down and away from your ears to release the muscles in your neck and shoulders.
- Do not hold your breath or you will impede your progress.

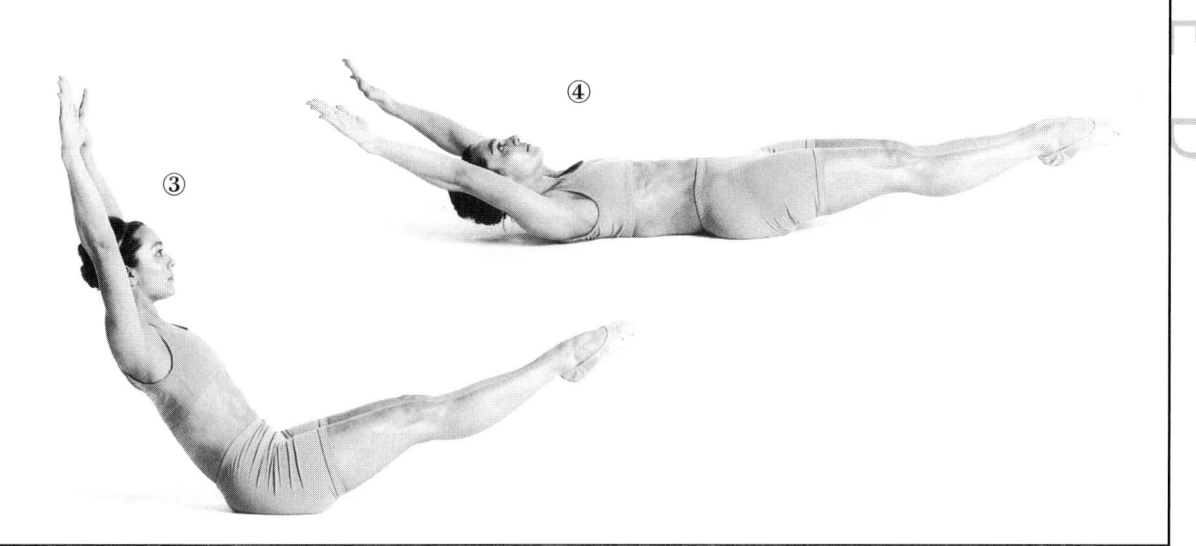

ADVANCED
HIP CIRCLES

Step by Step

1. Balance on your tailbone with your legs held in the V position of the Teasers, stretch your arms behind you, and place the palms of your hands on the mat behind you.
2. Inhale and move your legs, still held in the Pilates stance, down and around to the right.
3. Exhale and complete the circle, bringing the legs to the left and back up to the starting V position.
4. *Imagine your hands are stuck in cement and you are unable to move your torso except to keep it lifting to the ceiling.*
5. Remember that your upper body is providing the counterbalance as the weight of your legs circles down and around, so you must *press your hands deeper into the cement as your weight shifts*.
6. Switch directions with each circle, inhaling as you begin the circle and exhaling as you complete it. Try to make your legs feel very light as they circle so that you can engage the hip and abdominal muscles and not the muscles of the thigh.
7. Complete three sets of Hip Circles and end by bringing your legs down to the mat and rolling onto your stomach with your arms outstretched in front of you to prepare for Swimming. . . .

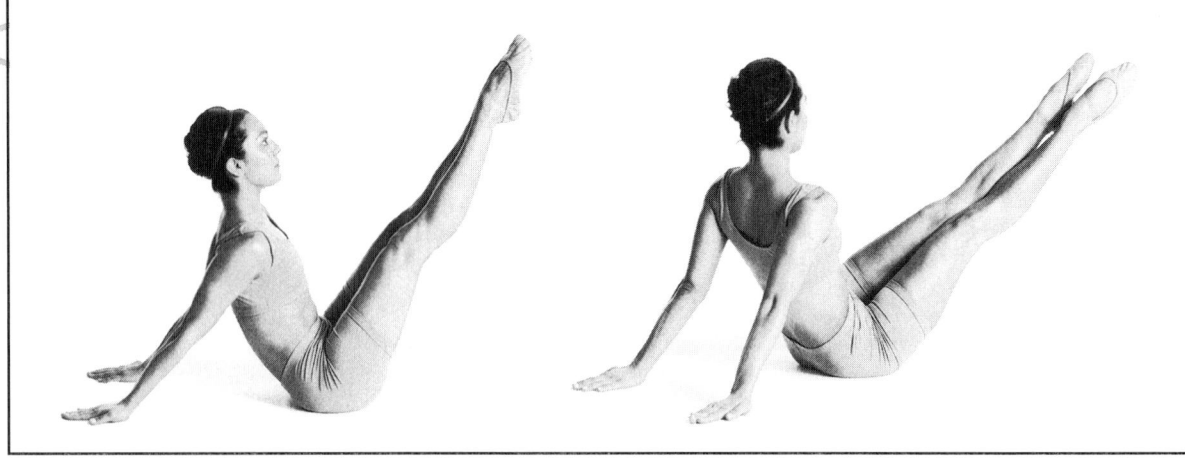

The Hip Circles focus on the muscles of the powerhouse and stretch the front of the shoulders, across the chest, and down the arms.

The Inside Scoop

Do not perform this exercise if you have a shoulder injury or a weak back.
If your back hurts, stop. Lie down and pull your knees into your chest to release your lower back.

- To maintain a rigid, lifted chest and straight arms as your legs circle.
- Think of pressing your chest up and away from the heels of your hands so as not to sink into your neck and back.
- The accent of the circles is on the upswing, so use all the power in your powerhouse to bring your legs back up to the center. Think of trying to bring your straight legs up to your nose.
- Press your shoulders down and away from your ears.
- Maintain a straight back with your ribs pulled in throughout.
- Do not allow your upper torso to move, or your neck to crane forward.
- Do not drop your legs below your point of control.
- Prop yourself up on your elbows if maintaining straight arms is too difficult.

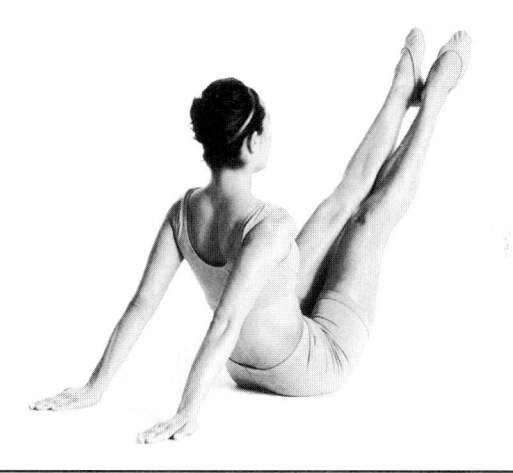

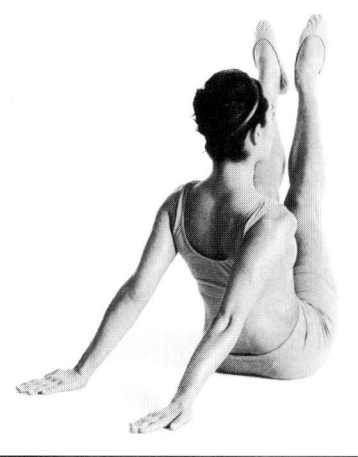

ADVANCED
SWIMMING

Step by Step

1. Lie on your stomach, completely outstretched on the mat, with your legs squeezing together behind you in the Pilates stance. Reach your fingertips for the wall in front of you.
2. Inhale, pulling your navel up into your spine as you bring your right arm and your left leg up into the air simultaneously. Hold them there as you lift your head and chest off the mat as well.
3. Switch the arms and legs by lifting your left arm and right leg above the mat.
4. Continue switching pairs until you have a swimming or light splashing motion in effect, inhaling for five counts and exhaling for five counts.
5. *Imagine you are balancing on a rock in the water and need to keep the movements controlled so you don't slip off.*
6. Complete two or three sets of five inhalations/exhalations each, and then sit back on your heels to release your lower back.
7. End by lying on your stomach with your hands placed palms down beneath your shoulders and your legs pressed together to go on to the Leg Pull Down. . . .

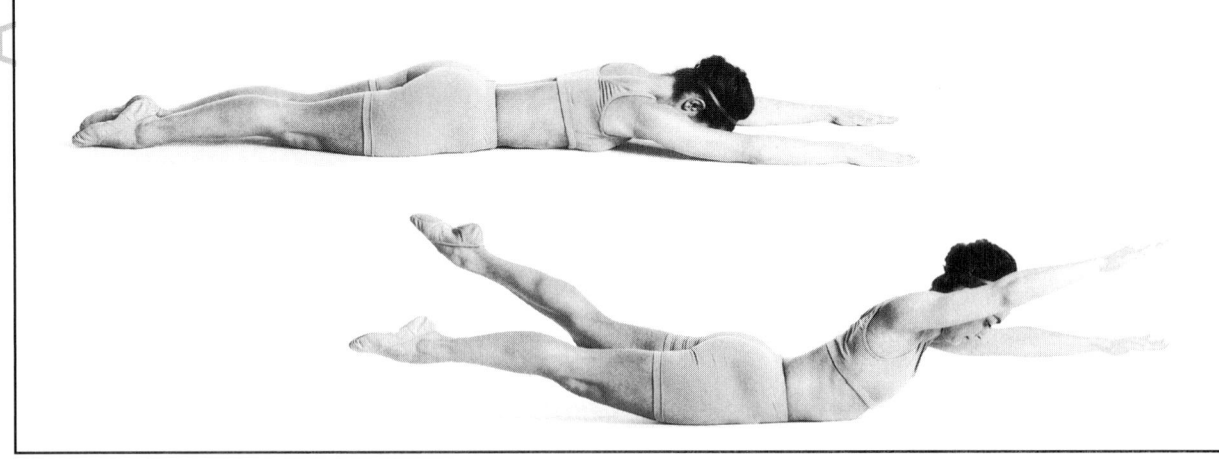

Swimming stretches and strengthens the muscles along your spine.

The Inside Scoop

GOAL
- To maintain a firm, lifted center throughout the swimming motion.

KEYS
- The key to the Swimming movement is to keep control from your center.
- Use your powerhouse to stay lifted, keeping your line of vision *above the surface of the water.*
- Remember to keep squeezing your buttocks together tightly to protect your lower back and to work the backs of your legs.
- Feel that you are stretching in opposition, fingers and toes reaching for the opposing walls of the room.
- Lengthen the back of your neck by pressing energy out of the crown of your head.
- Keep your arms and legs as straight as possible throughout the exercise without allowing them to touch the mat in between lifts.
- Make sure that your chest and thighs are lifted off the mat throughout.

NO-NOS
- Do not allow your limbs to drop as you perform the swimming motion.
- Do not allow your belly to drop or you will immediately feel this in your lower back!
- Do not allow your neck to crane backward.

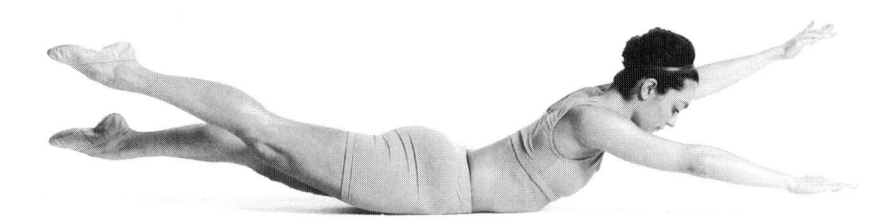

ADVANCED
THE LEG PULL-DOWN

Step by Step

1. Place your hands, palms down, onto the mat underneath your shoulders and pull your navel up into your spine as you press yourself up into a push-up position.
2. Squeeze up the back of your legs and make sure your body is held in a straight line, as if there were a steel rod from your head to your heel.
3. Shift your body weight backward, pressing your heels toward the mat, then rock forward onto the balls of your feet. *Imagine you are suspended by a cord leading from your belly button to the ceiling.*
4. Do this two or three times to warm up the tendons, then inhale as you lift one leg straight off the mat behind you and hold it there as you exhale and repeat the rocking movement.
5. Switch legs with each breath sequence.
6. Complete three sets and then flip onto your backside to perform the Leg Pull-Up. . . .

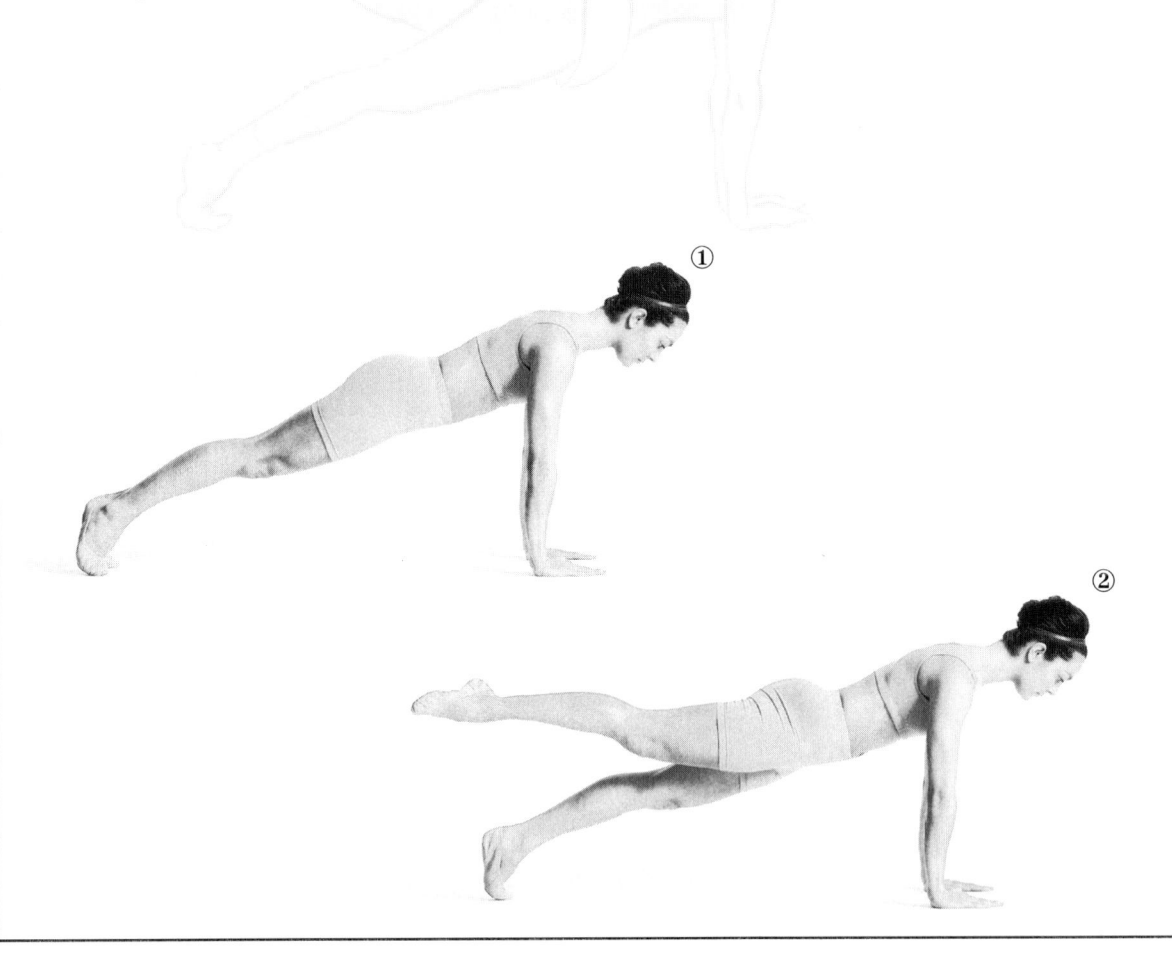

The Leg Pull-Down stretches the Achilles tendon (back of the ankle) and your calves, and stabilizes the powerhouse.

The Inside Scoop

GOAL

- To maintain a rigid center throughout the movement. (The movement is *like that of a battering ram being pulled back and rocked forward.* Think of the crown of your head as the contact point.)

KEYS

- Keep your arms and legs completely straight throughout the movement and think of pushing up and away from the heels of your hands so you do not sink into your wrists.
- Make sure you keep your navel firmly pulled up into your spine.
- Keep your neck long and your head aligned with your spine.

NO-NOS

- Do not allow your head to hang down.
- Do not allow your belly to hang out as gravity will want it to do.
- Do not twist in your hips as you lift your leg.

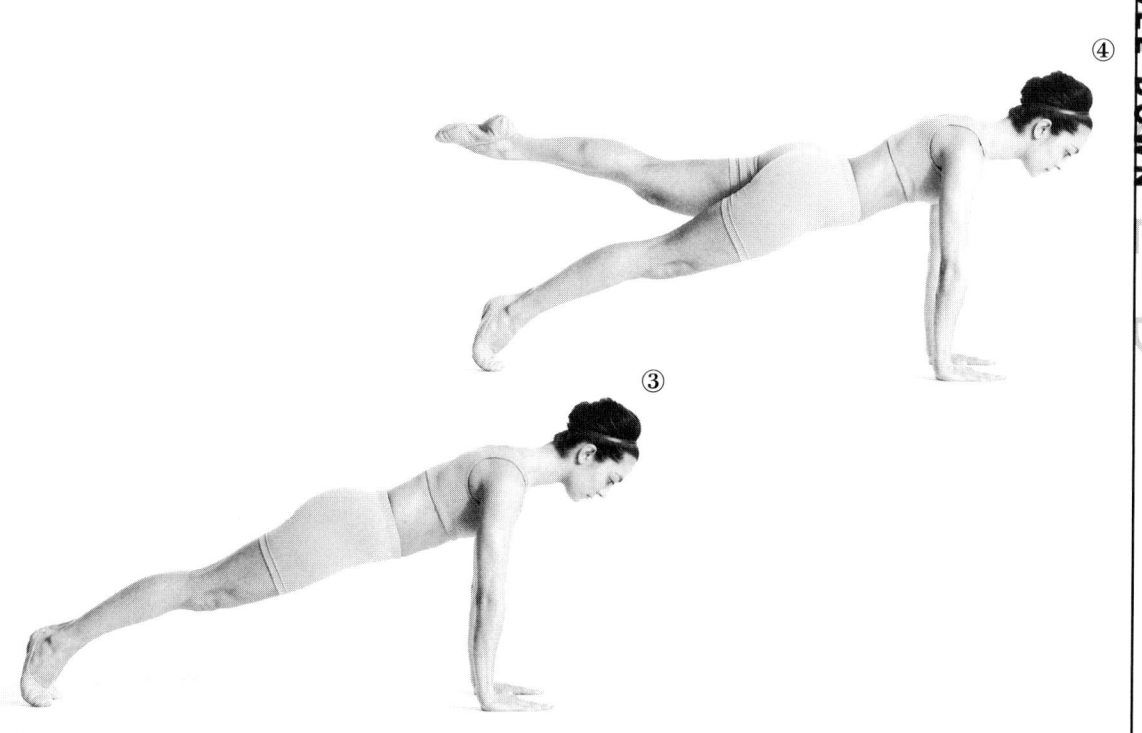

ADVANCED
LEG PULL-UP

Step by Step

1. Sit tall with your palms on the mat by your sides.
2. Lift your hips off the mat and firm your center with your legs long and squeezing together.
3. With straight arms and toes pointing to the mat, inhale and kick one leg straight up as high as possible without breaking at the waist.
4. Flex your foot at the height of the kick and exhale as you slowly lower your leg, pressing out of your heel.
5. As your heel nears the mat, point your toe and kick the leg up again, inhaling as you go.
6. *Imagine you are suspended by a sling around your hips that keeps your center lifted and still.*
7. Repeat the motion three times and then repeat with your other leg.
8. End by lowering your buttocks to the mat. Take a kneeling position with your knees aligned with the front edge of your mat and go on to the Kneeling Side Kicks. . . .

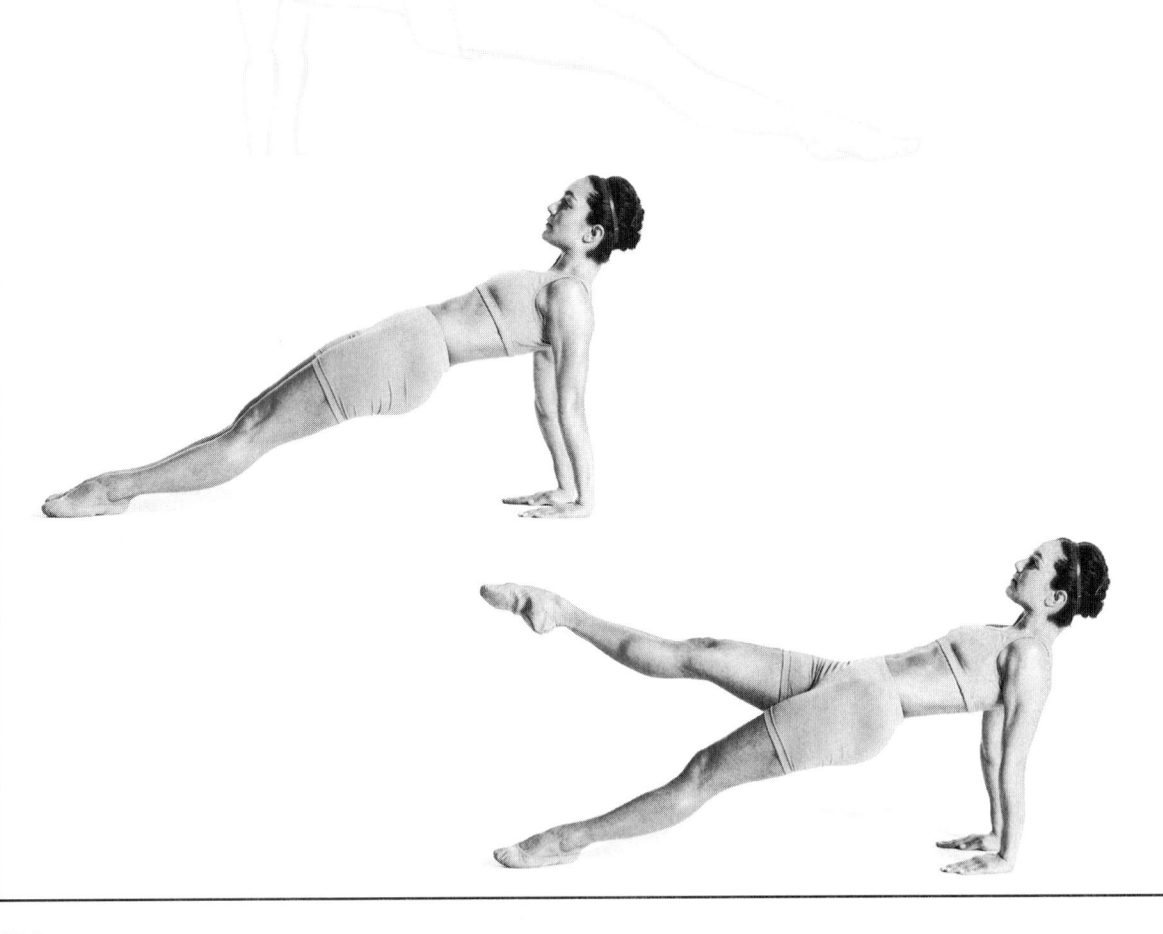

The Leg Pull-Up focuses on your powerhouse with emphasis on the buttocks. It also works the arms and shoulders and provides a stretch in the hamstrings.

The Inside Scoop

If you have a bad wrist or shoulder, leave this exercise out.

- To maintain a rigid, lifted center throughout the movements.
- Make sure your arms remain straight and you are pushing up off the heels of your hands so as not to sink into your wrists and shoulders.
- Keep your hips lifted at all times *as if there were a large, sharp pin beneath your buttocks.*
- Remember to keep your navel pulled firmly into your spine so that your belly does not push outward as you kick.
- Do not sink into your neck and shoulders.
- Your legs must remain straight at all times during this exercise. Do not bend at the knee or you will not be working from the hip and buttock as intended.
- Let your chin rest forward on your chest. As you progress, try to keep your head and neck aligned with your spine.

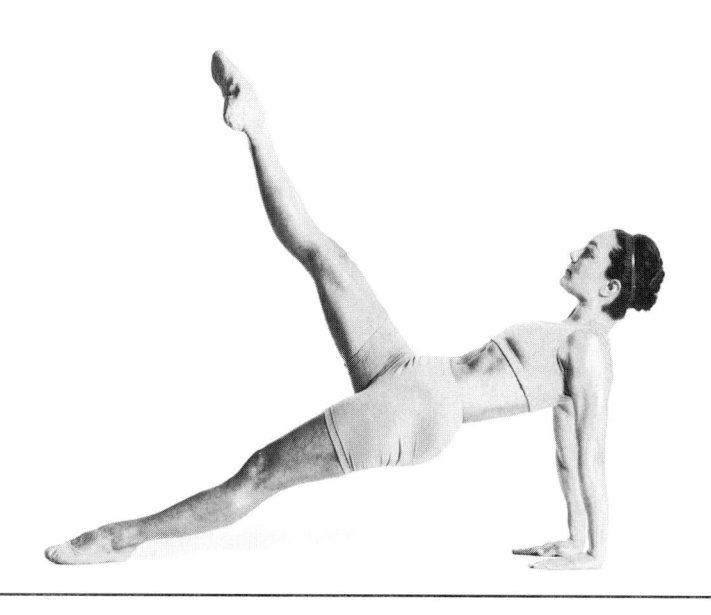

ADVANCED
KNEELING SIDE KICKS

Step by Step

1. Kneeling on the front edge of your mat, place one palm down on the mat directly under your shoulder and in alignment with your hips, fingers parallel to the mat.
2. Place your other hand behind your head with your elbow to the ceiling.
3. Straighten your top leg out along the mat in line with your body, making sure that your torso is grounded and your center is firm.
4. Lift your outstretched leg up off the mat as close to hip height as you can manage and balance. *Imagine you are suspended from the ceiling by a sling around your waist.*
5. Inhale as you kick your leg to the front wall, making sure you are not breaking in the waist as you go. *Imagine kicking a ball suspended before you.*
6. Exhale and swing your leg back, stretching it as far as you can without rocking in your hips or pushing your belly forward.
7. *Imagine the crown of your head is pressed into a wall and cannot move as you perform the kicking motions.*
8. Complete four sets of kicks on one side and then repeat the sequence balancing on your opposite side.

    NOTE: For an even more advanced challenge, try performing some of the other Side Kick variations from pages 98–115 while balanced in the kneeling position.

9. End by lowering your hip down to the mat and bringing your heels in toward your buttocks. Remain resting on one hand and go on to the Mermaid. . . .

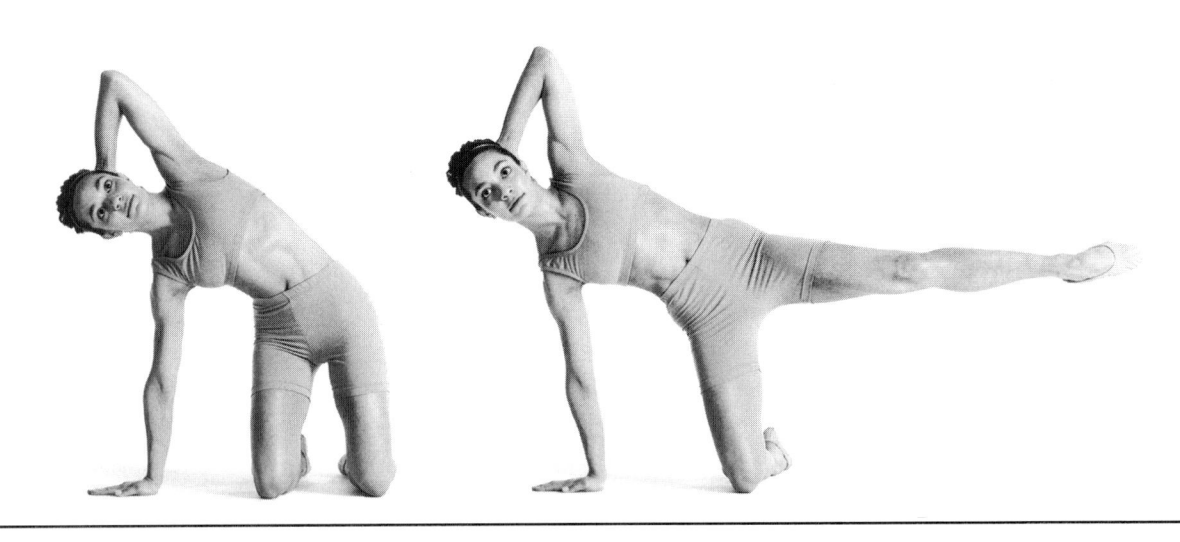

The Kneeling Side Kicks concentrate on the waistline and hips. Emphasis is also on balance and coordination.

The Inside Scoop

If you have a bad knee, leave this exercise out. The Kneeling Side Kicks are essentially the Side Kicks (pages 98–115) performed balancing on one knee. Use similar images, where helpful, to master the movements.

- To remain perfectly still and rigid in your upper body as you perform the kicks.

- Keep your elbow to the ceiling so that your shoulder and chest remain open throughout the exercise.
- Keep your navel pulled firmly to your spine and your hips still as you go.
- Keep your head lifted and aligned with your spine.

- Do not sink into your neck or shoulders.

- Start with small kicks front and back and concentrate instead on your balance and control before engaging in big movements. Once you are able to remain still in your torso as you kick your leg, begin making the kicks stronger to challenge yourself.

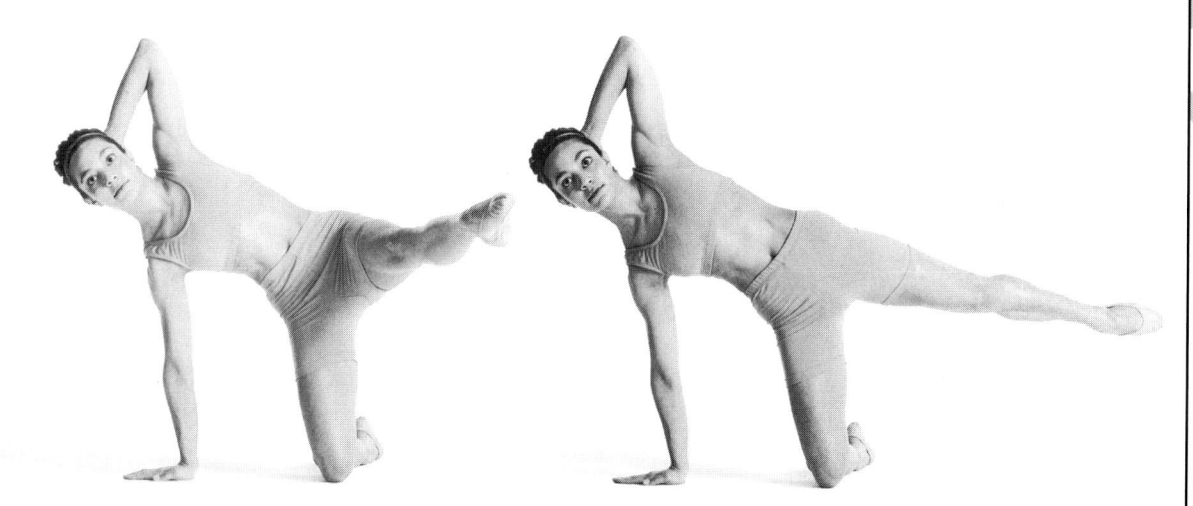

ADVANCED

MERMAID/SIDE BENDS

Step by Step

1. Sit on one side with your knees slightly bent and together, your top foot on the mat just in front of the other.
2. Place your hand, palm down and parallel to the mat, directly beneath your shoulder. Allow your top hand to rest on your shin.
3. Press up onto a straight arm and bring your upper foot to rest on top of the other. You should be balanced on your hand and the side of your foot with your body lifted and straight, aligned from head to toe. *Imagine you are suspended at your hips by a sling attached to the ceiling.*
4. Turn your head toward the ceiling and try to bring your chin down to your top shoulder. Stretching your arm and fingertips down toward your feet, exhale slowly and allow for a slight dip in your hips. You should feel a stretch up the underside of your body.
5. Inhale deeply and lift your arm up and straight overhead alongside your ear, reaching as far away from your feet as possible. Allow for a lift in your hips and return your head to a position in line with your spine. You should now feel a stretch along the top side of your body.
6. Repeat the movements three times and then lower your hip to the mat, take hold of your ankles with your top hand, and bring your supporting arm overhead, bending toward your legs to stretch your side in a mermaid pose. Switch to the other side.
7. End by lowering your hips to the mat and then sitting tall with your legs extended out in front of you and your palms resting on the mat by your sides to prepare for the Boomerang. . . .

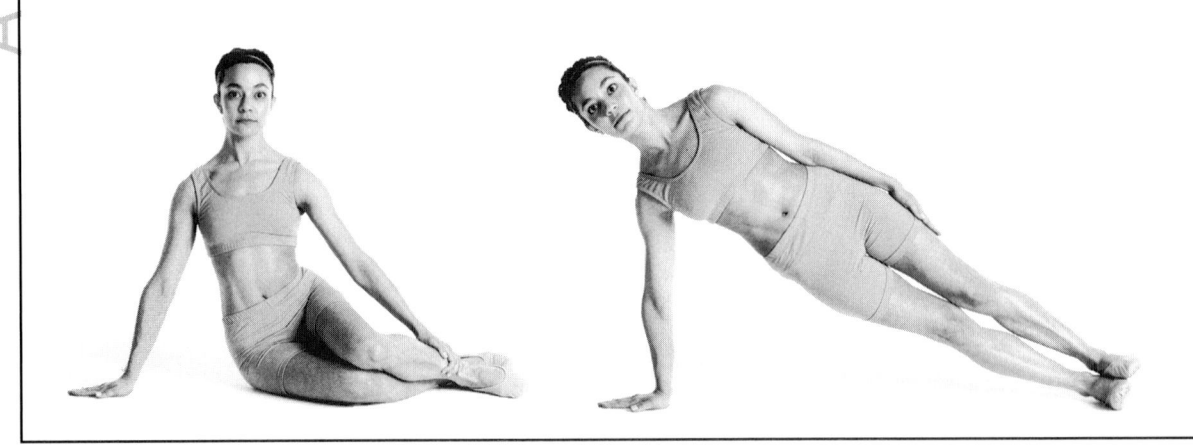

The Mermaid concentrates on the muscles of the arms, shoulders, and wrists. It also stretches the hips and waistline and helps to develop balance.

The Inside Scoop

If you have a bad wrist or shoulder, leave this exercise out.

- To maintain a rigid body and perfect balance throughout.

- The key to this exercise is remaining lifted out of your shoulder throughout the movement.
- Stay firm in your center and lifted in your hips.
- Keep the movements slow and controlled to facilitate balance.

- Do not allow your body weight to sink into your wrist and shoulder.
- Keep your arm directly alongside your ear as you stretch overhead. Do not pitch your body forward as you go.

- As this is a difficult postion to maintain, try to map out the motion before pressing up onto your arm. Practice stretching your arm and turning your head while your hips are still resting on the mat. When you feel confident, try just holding the lifted position and balancing there for a breath. Finally, put the movements together to perform the full exercise.

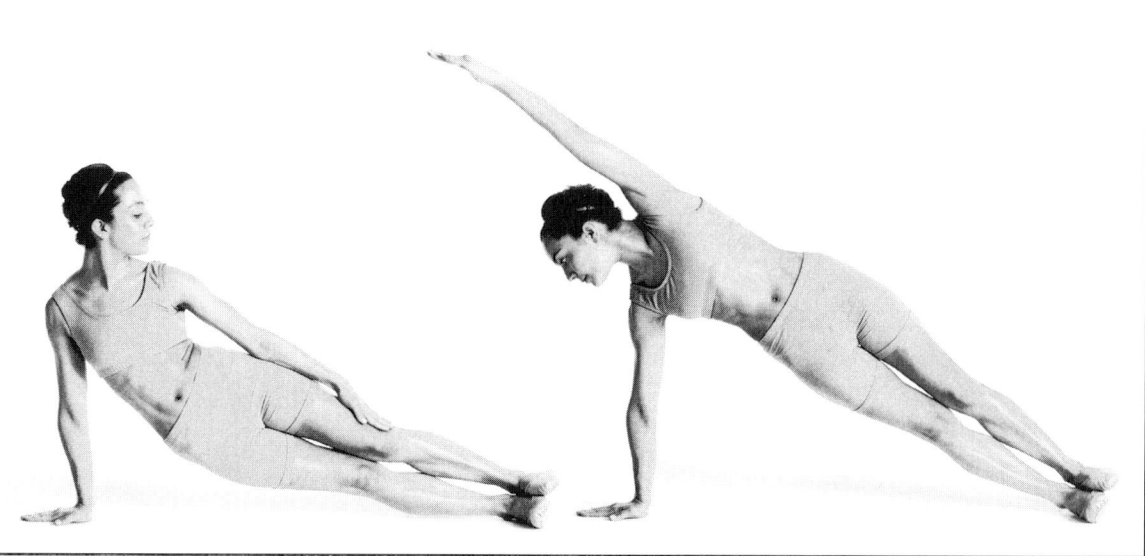

ADVANCED
THE BOOMERANG

Step by Step

1. Sit tall with straight legs and cross your right ankle over your left. Press your hands into the mat on either side of your body to help you lift up out of your hips.
2. Inhale and roll back until your legs are overhead. Do not roll onto your neck.
3. Hold this position steady, exhaling as you open and close your legs in a snapping motion, recrossing your ankles, now with the left over right.
4. Inhale and roll up into your V position, bringing your arms forward to your toes.
5. Balancing in this position, bring your arms down and around the sides of your body, clasping them together behind your back and stretching them away from your torso.
6. Slowly, and with great control, exhale and begin leaning forward until your legs touch the mat and your nose is on your knees in a deep bow.
7. Keeping your arms lifted behind you, gently unclasp your hands and circle them forward to your toes.
8. Complete two sets (or four Boomerangs), switching ankles each time. End by sitting up and lifting your bottom forward to your heels to prepare for the Seal.

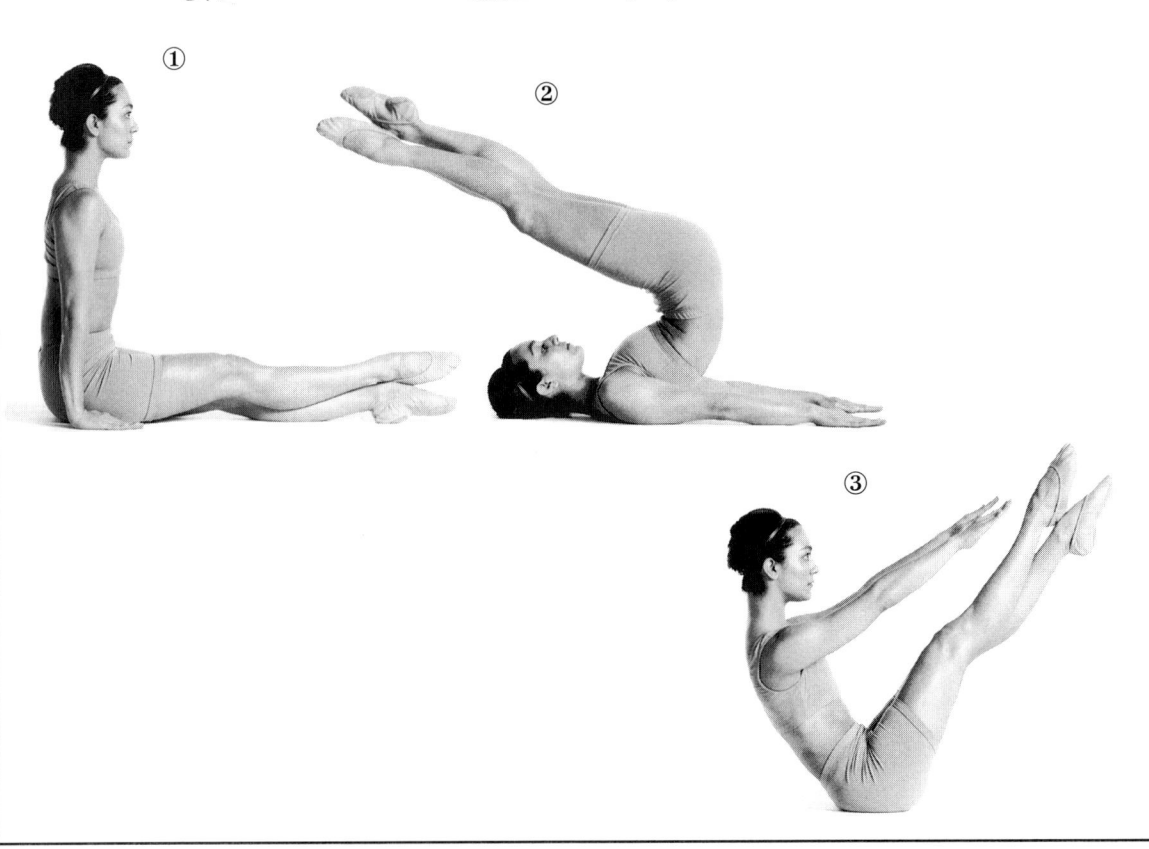

The Boomerang is one of the most comprehensive exercises of the matwork. It stretches and strengthens almost all the muscles of your body.

The Inside Scoop

This exercise can seem intimidating at first, but if you use the imagery from the Rollover and Teasers to help find your focus, you'll get it in no time.

- Initiate from your powerhouse, keeping your body stiff so your movements do not get sloppy.
- Keep your arms as straight as possible and push off your palms as you lift your legs.
- Balance your weight on the back of your shoulders as you recross your ankles.
- If you are very flexible in your shoulders, do not lift your arms so high behind you that your shoulders pop. Keep the movements controlled at all times.
- Let your neck relax as you stretch forward over your legs but do not relax so long as to interrupt the dynamic flow of the exercise sequence.

- Do not roll onto your neck.
- Do not allow your legs to drop down to the mat after balancing in the Teaser position. Think of "floating" forward as you slowly lower your legs and torso with control.

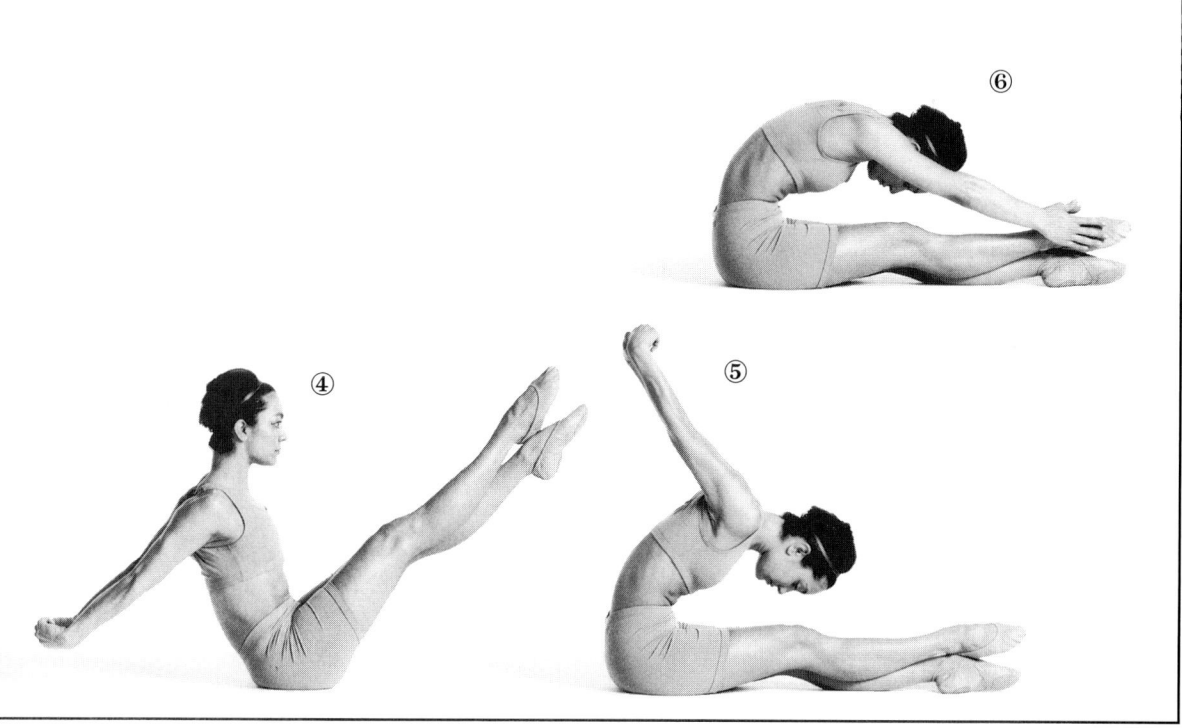

BEGINNER

THE SEAL

Step by Step

1. Sit at the front of your mat with your knees bent to your chest and heels together. Open your knees to shoulder width and slide a hand under and around each ankle. Pull your feet up off the mat until you are balancing on your tailbone.
2. Inhale and press your navel deeper into your spine.
3. Roll back, pulling your feet with you. Do not roll too far onto the back of your neck. Balance on the back of the shoulders instead, allowing your legs to extend slightly until your feet are over your head.
4. Balancing in the backward position, clap your heels together three times *like a seal clapping its flippers.*
5. Exhale as you roll forward, tucking your chin into your chest. Pull on your ankles to come up.
6. Balance in the forward position and clap your heels together three times.
7. *Imagine you are on rockers, balancing on the edges both front and back and trying not to tip over in either direction.*
8. Repeat the sequence six times, allowing yourself to feel the massage up and down the muscles of your back.
9. For an advanced transitional challenge: Begin building momentum as you are nearing completion of your sixth repetition. Cross your ankles while in the backward position, release your hands, and roll up and forward into a standing position. Use your powerhouse and the dynamic of your arms reaching out in front of you to bring you up.

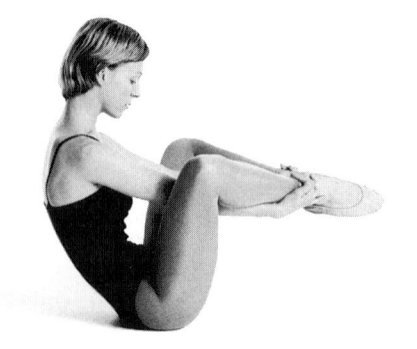

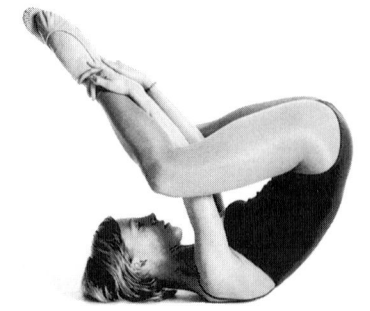

The Seal massages the spinal muscles, works the powerhouse, and tests balance and coordination.

The Inside Scoop

If you have a bad neck, leave this exercise out.

- To be able to balance, both back and forward, with your feet only a few inches from the mat in both positions.
- The key to the Seal is remembering to relax and enjoy the movement. This exercise is playfully called the "dessert" exercise of the matwork because it feels so good after all the hard work you have done.
- Use the control of your powerhouse and breath to bring you forward and back.
- Allow your legs to straighten slightly as you bring them overhead, but leave your hips down.
- Do not throw your head back and forth to accomplish the rocking motion of this exercise. Initiate the movements from your powerhouse and use the pulling on your ankles to help build momentum as you begin.
- Do not roll too far onto your neck. You should remain with your weight resting on the back of your shoulders instead.
- This should be a relaxing motion, so do not tense your shoulders or legs as you roll.
- If it is too difficult to master the clapping movement of the feet in the backward position, simply leave it out and clap the feet only on the forward balance portion.

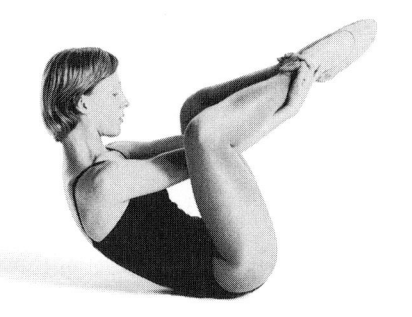

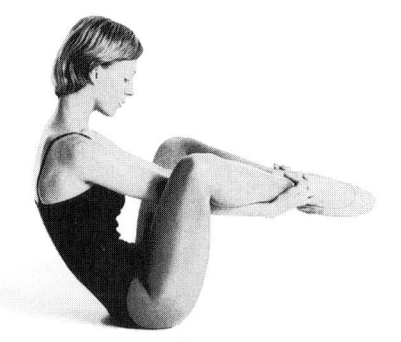

ADVANCED
PUSH-UPS

Step by Step

1. Stand at the back of your mat with your feet and legs in the Pilates stance.
2. Inhale deeply and pull your navel into your spine.
3. Exhale and walk your hands down the front of your legs until your palms are pressing into the mat. Allow for the stretch up the backs of your legs.
4. Inhale and walk your hands out on the mat until your palms are directly beneath your shoulders.
5. Exhale and lower your hips until they are in line with the rest of your body. *Imagine you are suspended by a heavy spring attached to your belt loops and up to the ceiling.*
6. Perform three Push-Ups by bending and straightening your arms with your elbows held tightly to your sides. (Breathe normally.)
7. On your last Push-Up, fold up in your center, bringing your chest toward your legs. Exhale as you press your palms and heels firmly into the mat and pull your navel up deeper into your spine for a complete stretch. *Imagine being pulled up in your center by the spring.*
8. Inhale and walk your hands back toward your feet. Keep your legs as straight as possible as you go.
9. Exhale and roll your body back up to a standing position.
10. Repeat the sequence no more than three times.

    NOTE: For an advanced challenge, try performing the entire Push-Up sequence while balancing on one leg. The same steps apply for the single-leg Push-Up, but remember to keep your back leg *lifted* throughout the entire exercise. Remember to repeat the sequence on the other leg for uniformity.

11. End by standing tall and proud. You have just finished the full Pilates Matwork sequence!

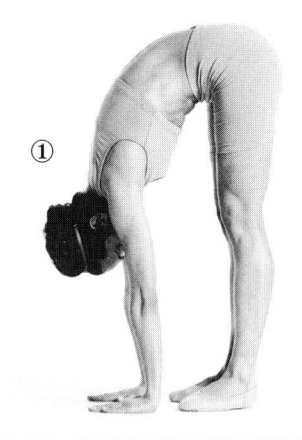

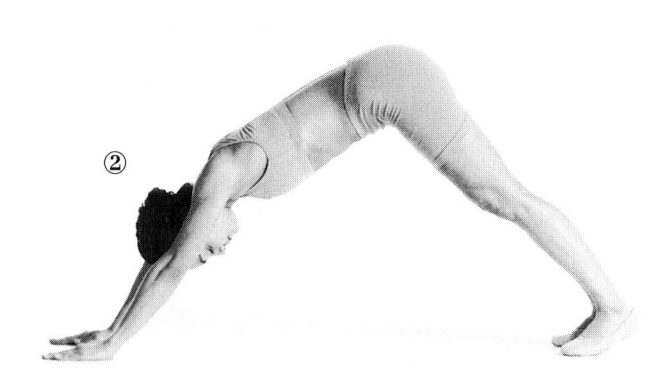

Push-Ups concentrate on the shoulders, chest, arms, and upper back. Pilates' Push-Ups also stretch your shoulders and hamstrings.

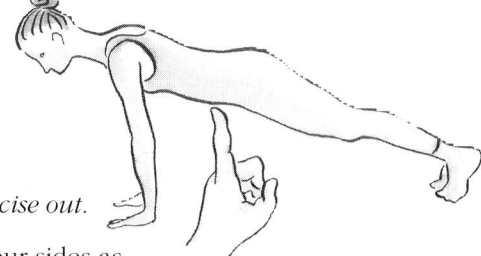

The Inside Scoop

If you have a bad wrist or shoulder, leave this exercise out.

- To keep your body rigid and elbows pinned to your sides as you perform the Push-Ups.

- The key to the Pilates Push-Up is maintaining a firm center, with navel to spine and your buttocks and legs squeezing firmly together behind you. Powerhouse!
- Maintain a straight line with your body and head. Think of trying to touch your chin to the mat as you lower your body, and push off the heels of your hands as you lift up.
- The more rigid you are able to keep your body, the less chance of collapsing in your center. Keep your movements small and progress slowly.

- Do not allow your middle to drop, as that places the majority of your body's weight onto your shoulders.
- Do not allow your head to hang as you perform the Push-Ups.

- If you find it too difficult to keep your elbows pinned into your sides, you may allow them to remain slightly open. Do not make a habit of this!

- As you walk your hands back toward your leg after the single leg push-up, lift your back leg higher and maintain that height as you try to lift both hands off the floor simultaneously. Rise, stretching your arms out long in front of you and your leg out long behind you, as in an arabesque. Bring your feet togther and stand tall before repeating the sequence with your other leg.

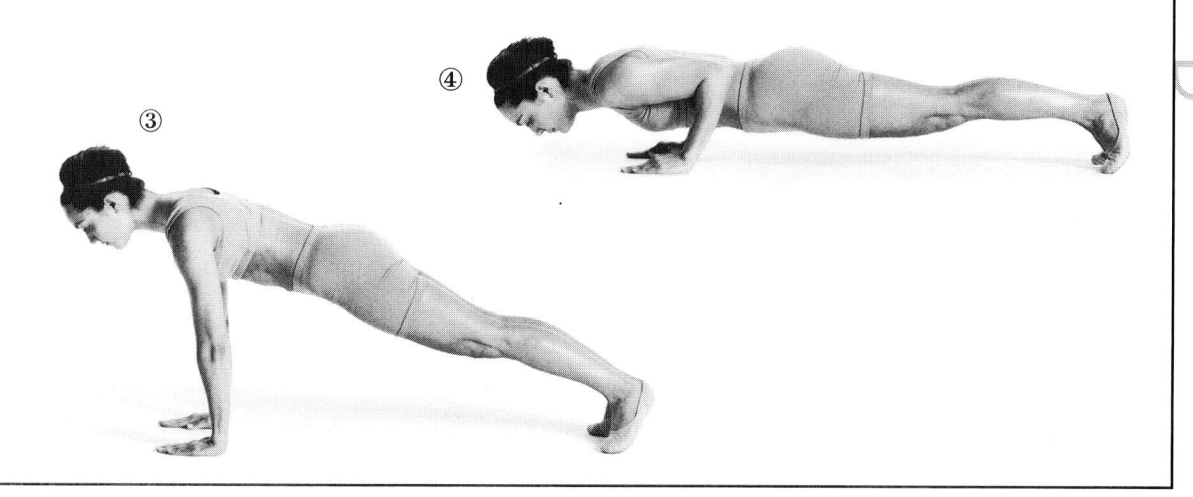

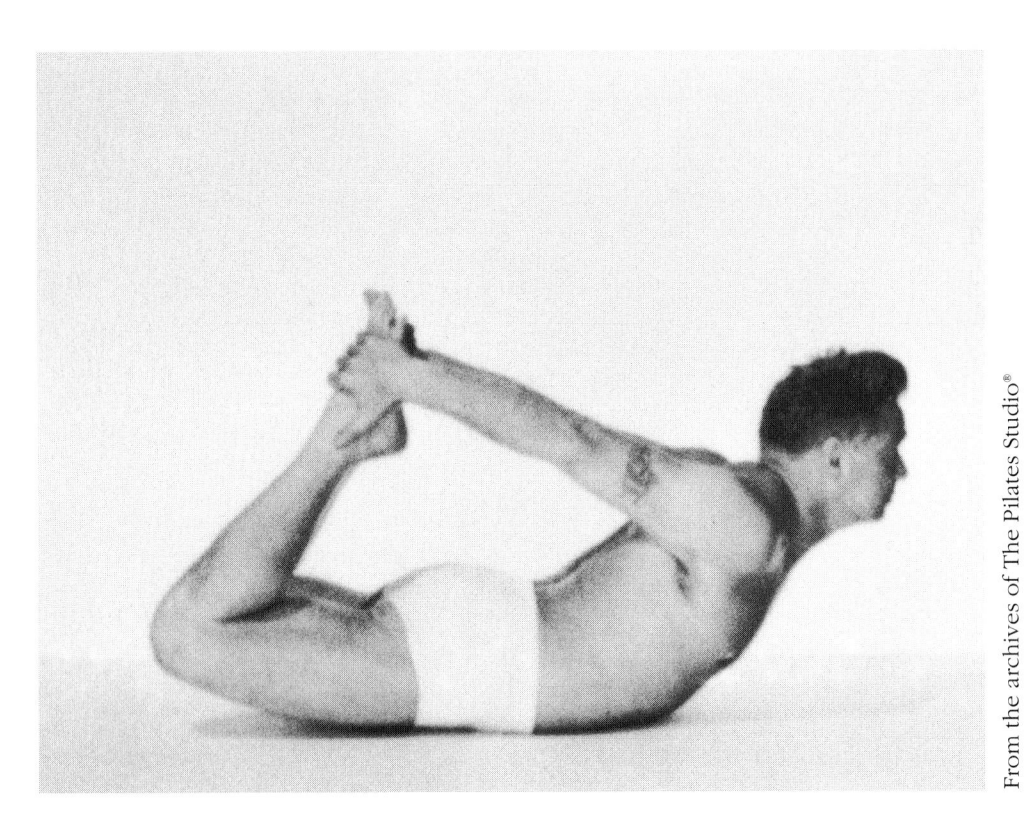

Joseph Pilates demonstrates "Rocking."

From the archives of The Pilates Studio®

Advanced Extras

These exercises are mostly adapted from the apparatus and are for the advanced student only.

1. Rowing III
2. Rowing IV
3. Rowing I
4. Twist I
5. Twist II
6. Rocking

ADVANCED EXTRA

ROWING III

Step by Step

1. Sit tall with your legs extended in front of you and squeeze them together. Feet are relaxed or softly pointed.
2. Bring your elbows into your sides and sit taller off the mat by squeezing your buttocks.
3. Inhale and reach your arms forward on an upward diagonal, lifting in your back but not in your shoulders.
4. Exhale and press your palms in a downward motion toward the floor *as if pressing down on a heavy lever*. Feel your shoulders also pressing down and away from your ears. Keep your chest lifted.
5. Inhale and bring your arms up above your head, just in front of your ears, without sinking into your back or shoulders.
6. Exhale and open your arms to the sides, pressing your palms downward *as if pushing down on two benches* by your sides. Make sure that your hands are still within your peripheral vision and that you are lifting in your back and chest.
7. Fold your elbows tightly back into your sides and repeat the sequence three to five times.
8. End by bringing your palms down to the mat alongside your hips and go on to Rowing IV. . . .

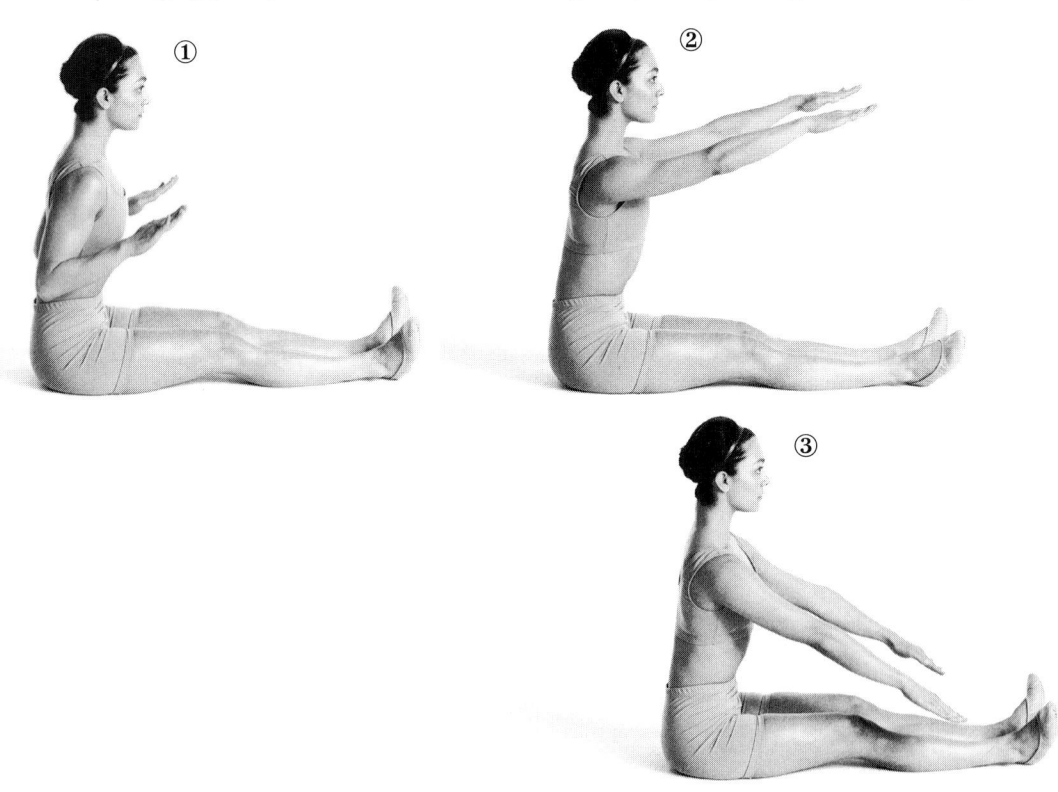

The Rowing exercises concentrate on posture and abdominal control. Their main focus is on the movements of the upper body, but stability in the lower body is essential to mastering the exercise.

The Extra Scoop

Although this exercise may feel like a simple circling of the arms, it is the way you perform the movement that counts!

- The challenge of this exercise is to remain completely still while lifting tall in your torso and cinching in your waist throughout the sequence.
- Squeeze your buttocks and legs together tightly in the Pilates stance throughout the movement.
- Keep your chest lifted and slightly in front of your hips so that you can stretch up and forward and not sink back into your tail.
- Make sure the back of your neck remains long and lifted from the crown of your head.
- Keep your shoulders pressing down and away from your ears to allow for a stretch in your neck.
- Do not allow your shoulders to creep up around your ears.

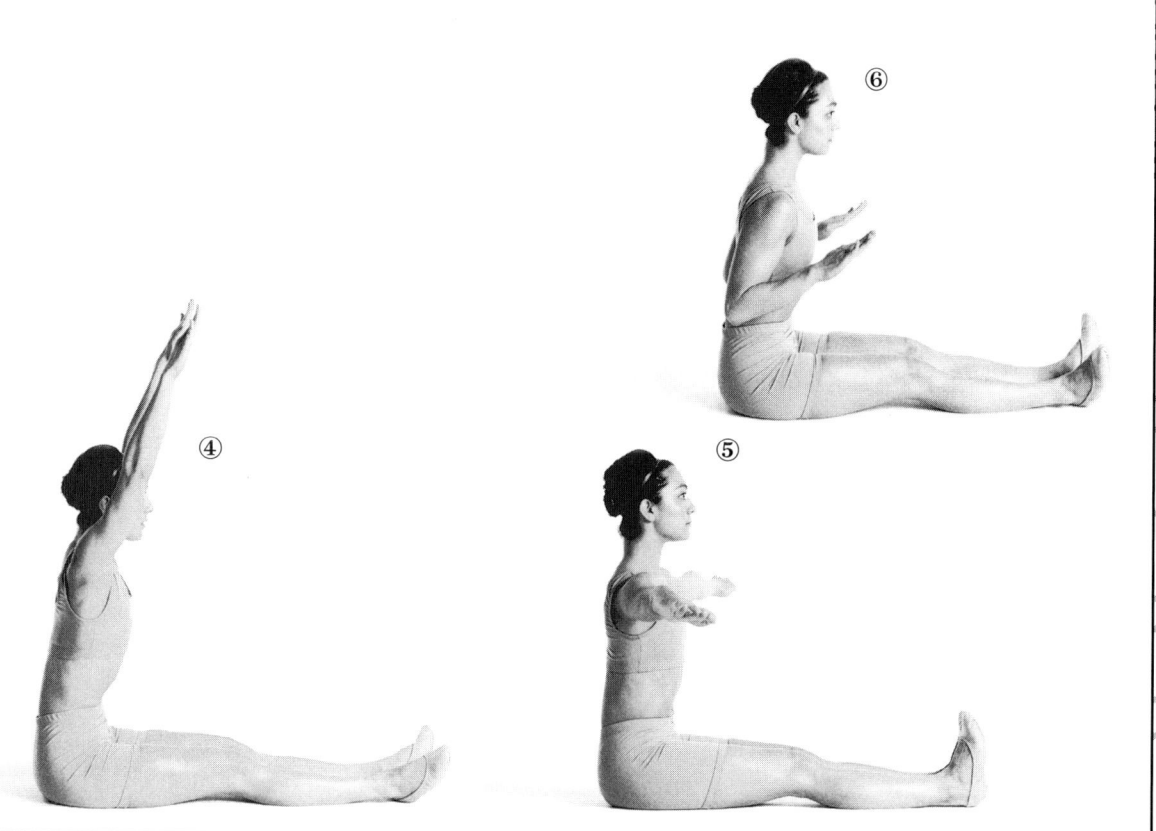

ADVANCED EXTRA

ROWING IV

Step by Step

1. Start by sitting tall with your legs extended in front of you, feet flexed (from your ankles, not your toes) and palms pressing into the mat by your sides.
2. Inhale, pulling your navel deep into your spine, and exhale as you fold your body in half, bringing your head and chest down to your legs.
3. Inhale and slide your hands along the mat past your heels. Keep pressing energy out of the heels.
4. Exhale as you slowly roll up to a sitting position, making sure you are lifting out of your back and waist and not from your shoulders. *Imagine pressing each vertebra into a wall* as you roll up to sitting. Your arms should now be held in midair parallel to your legs.
5. Inhale as you lift your arms up overhead. Stop just before your ears and stretch taller, keeping your feet flexed and pressing long out of your heels.
6. Exhale and open your arms to the sides, pressing your palms downward *as if pressing down on two benches* by your sides. Remember to keep your hands within your peripheral vision as you bring them down to the mat.
7. Inhale and then fold in half, repeating the sequence three to five times.
8. End by sitting tall with your hands drawn into your breastbone to prepare for Rowing I. . . .

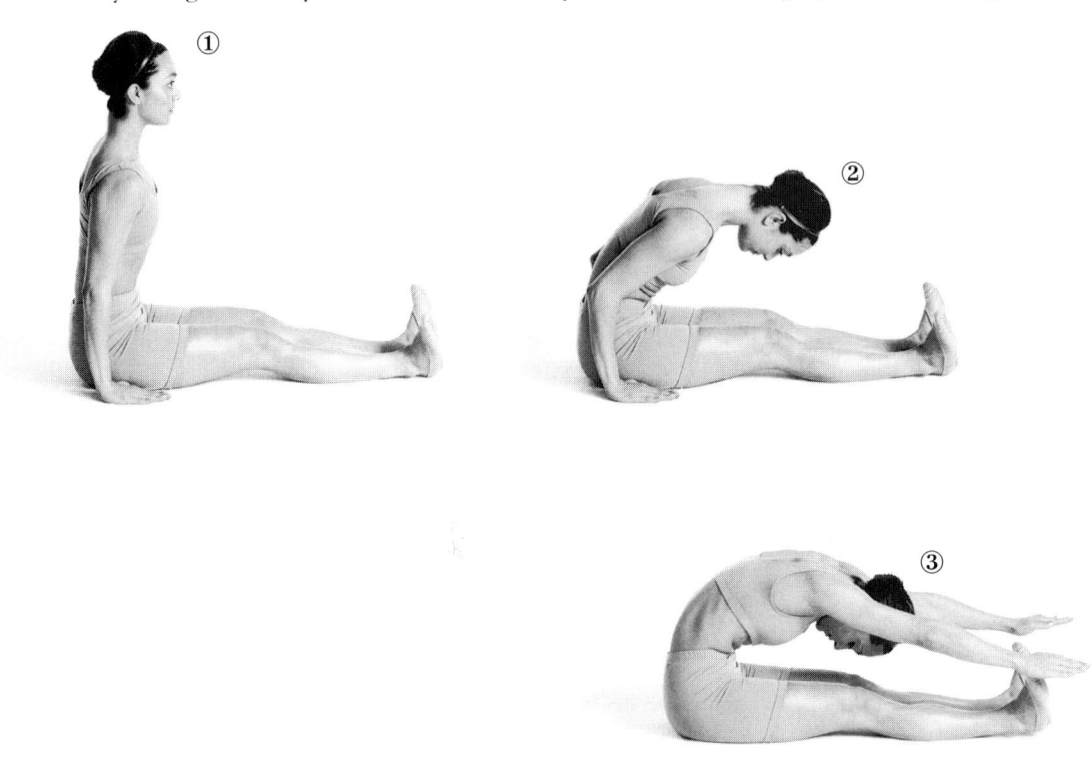

This exercise works your powerhouse, stretches your back and hamstrings, and improves posture.

The Extra Scoop

GOAL
- To stay lifted and long in your waist and lower back throughout the arm movements.

KEYS
- Fluidity! Allow yourself to feel the fluid movements as you perform them.
- Press your palms down into the mat as you slide them past your heels to engage your abdominals.
- Keep stretching forward as you roll up. *Imagine you are inflating with air.*
- Stay pitched slightly forward in your hips to keep your powerhouse engaged. Navel to spine!
- Squeeze your buttocks and legs tightly together in the Pilates stance throughout the movements.
- Push your heels away from you as you roll up.

NO-NOS
- Do not roll up from your head or shoulders.
- Do not sit back on your tail as you roll up to a tall seated position.
- Do not lift in your shoulders as you circle your arms overhead.

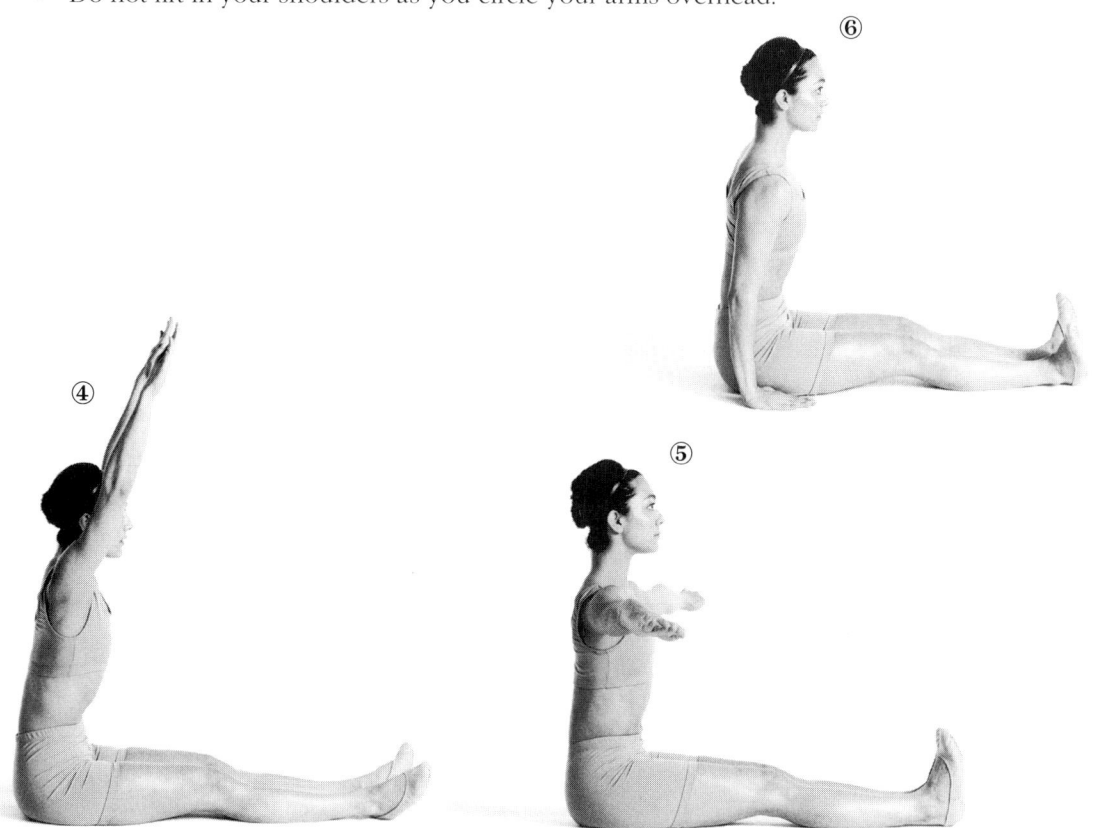

ADVANCED EXTRA

ROWING I

Step by Step

1. Sit tall with your legs extended in front of you, feet flexed and your hands, made into fists, pulled into your breastbone. Extend your elbows without raising your shoulders.
2. Inhale as you roll your upper body backward, scooping your belly down toward the mat and squeezing your buttocks and the backs of your inner thighs together tightly for stability.
4. Holding yourself steady with your powerhouse, open your arms out wide to your sides with your palms facing back behind you.
5. Exhale and bring your upper body through your arms. *Imagine you are pressing your palms back into a wall,* and stretch down toward your legs. Allow your hands to clasp at your tailbone as you stretch forward.
6. Inhale and slowly lift your joined hands upward, stretching your arms toward the ceiling. Do not allow your shoulders to over rotate or dislocate (pop out of the joint) as you go.
7. Slowly unclasp your hands and exhale as you circle your arms around to your feet in a controlled sweeping motion. Visualize the arm movement of the butterfly stroke in swimming as you perform this motion.
8. Roll up to a straight-backed sitting position, drawing your hands back into your breastbone, and repeat the sequence three to five times.

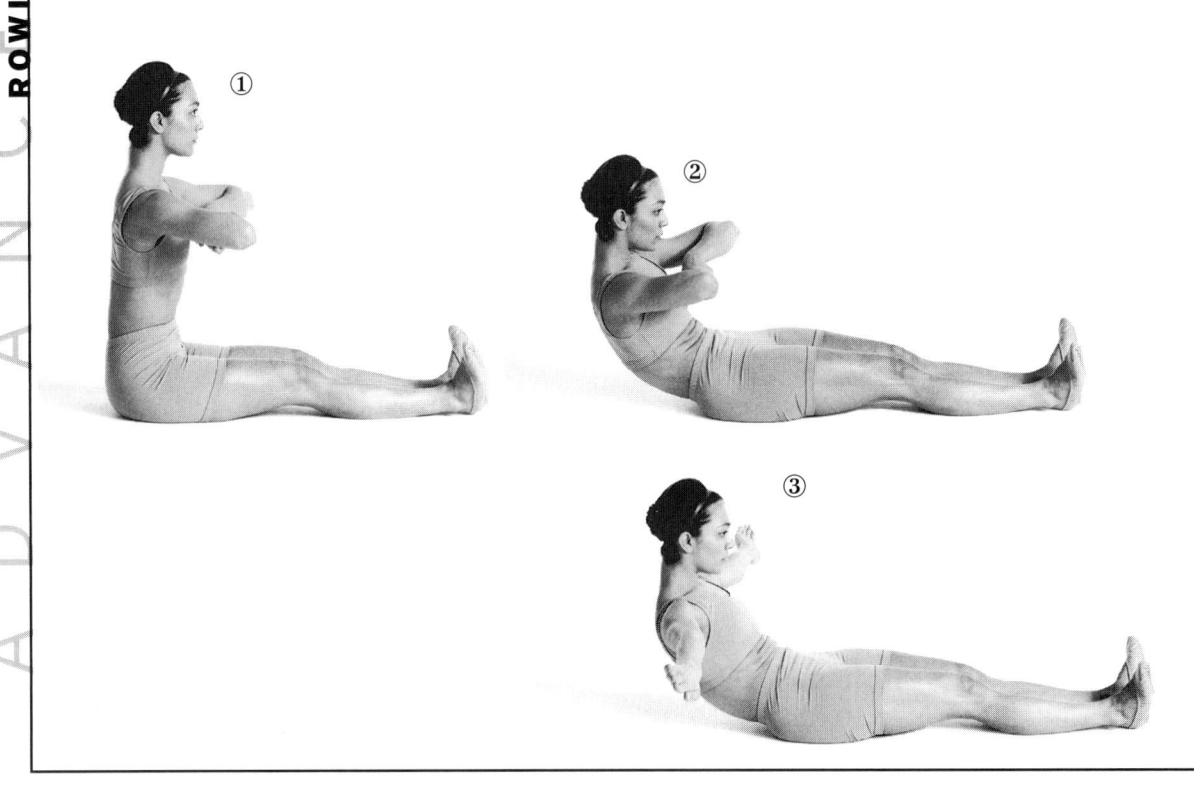

This exercise works your powerhouse while stretching your arms, back, shoulders, and hamstrings. It improves balance and tests your muscle control.

The Extra Scoop

- To stay lengthened out of your lower back throughout the movements of the rowing.
- *Imagine you are pulling on springs attached to the wall in front of you.*
- Keep your buttocks and legs squeezing together tightly in the Pilates stance throughout.
- Keep your heels firmly planted on the mat in front of you.
- Navel to spine!
- Create resistance as you press your arms back and stretch forward.

- Do not roll so far back as to lose control of your powerhouse, or tip backward.
- Do not let your shoulders creep up around your ears.
- Do not flop forward over your legs. Pull back in your powerhouse to enhance the stretch.
- Do not allow your shoulders to overrotate in the socket.

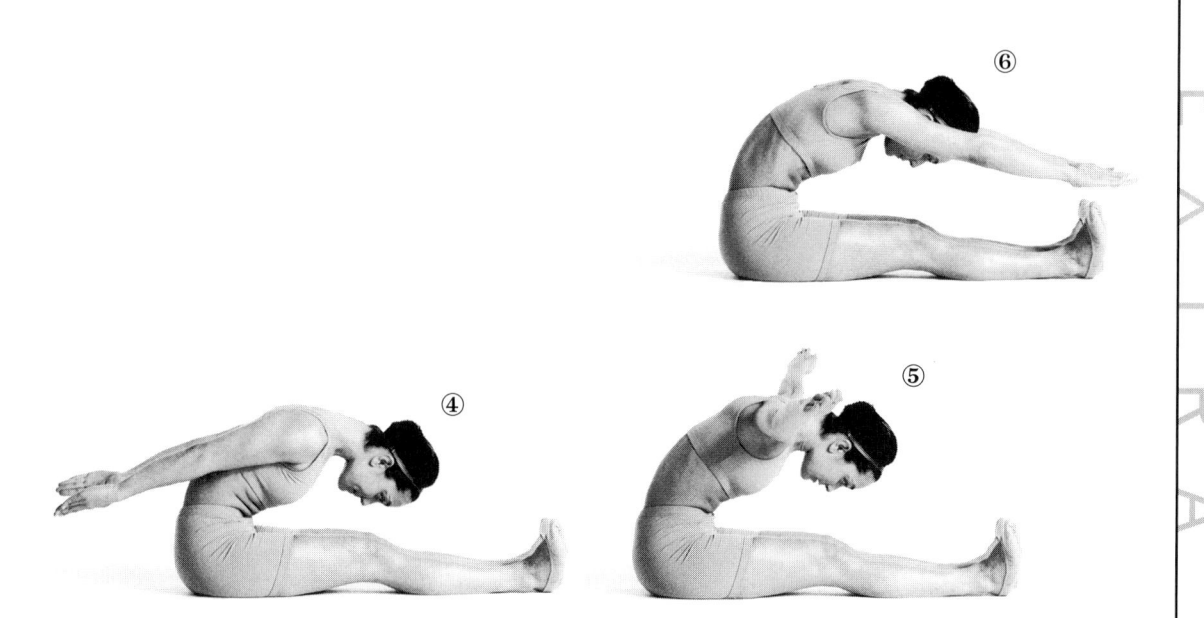

ADVANCED EXTRA

TWIST I

Step by Step

1. Sit on the side of one hip, propped up on a straight arm, fingers facing away from you.
2. Bend your knees and cross your top foot over your bottom foot. Hold your ankles in close to your bottom with your top hand and lean slightly into your supporting hand.
3. In one motion pull your navel up into your spine, inhaling, and lift your bottom hip to the ceiling by straightening your legs. *Imagine you are being pulled by a sling around your center.*
4. As your bottom hip lifts behind you, bring your top arm up and overhead. *Imagine drawing a sweeping arc up and over your body.*
5. Keep your eyes focused on your supporting hand throughout and lengthen your neck by stretching from the crown of your head. Reach your top arm long out of your side.
6. Reverse the motion of the twist, returning your bottom hip to the mat in a slow, controlled movement. Focus on stretching your arm up and away from your body as you lower yourself down.
7. Complete three controlled twists and then switch sides, working your opposite hip for three more.

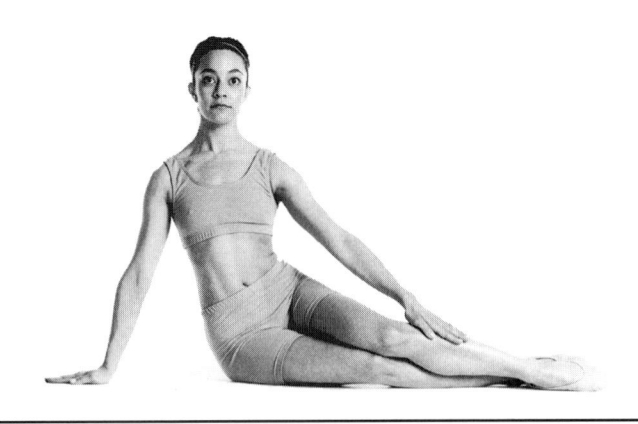

This extra works your abdominals, arms, and waistline; stretches the side of your body; and improves balance and coordination.

The Extra Scoop

GOAL
- To keep your body perfectly steady throughout the twisting movement.

KEYS
- Keep lifting your bottom hip to the ceiling and reaching your top arm away to increase the stretch up the side of your body.
- Lift your belly up and away from your supporting arm to relieve the pressure on your wrist.
- Actively stretch the crown of your head away from your body to support your neck.

NO-NO
- Do not sink into your shoulders or wrists at any time during the sequence.

PROGRESSION
- The closer you bring your supporting arm to your body, the harder the exercise will become.

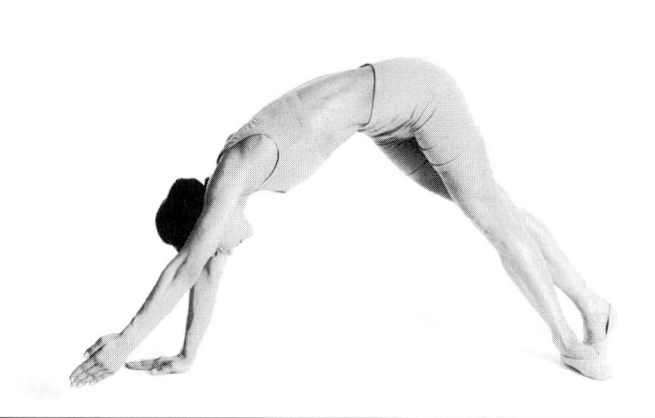

ADVANCED EXTRA
TWIST II

Step by Step

1. Sit on one side with your knees slightly bent and together, your top foot on the mat just in front of the other.
2. Place your hand, palm down and fingers facing away from you, almost directly beneath your shoulder. Allow your top hand to rest on your knee.
3. In one movement press up onto a straight arm and straighten your legs, bringing your top arm up and overhead until it is alongside your ear. Look toward your outstretched hand.
4. You should be balanced on your hand and the sides of your feet with your body lifted and straight, aligned from head to toe. *Imagine you are suspended by a strong spring attached through your belt loops and up to the ceiling.*
5. Maintaining your balance, bring your top arm down and thread it through the space between your lifted body and the floor. Allow your head and upper body to slowly follow, twisting to face the mat without allowing your hips to move.
6. Now take your arm out and reach it back, allowing your upper body to twist toward the ceiling.
7. Return to your long, aligned position of Step 4. Then, bringing your arm around and down, slowly lower your hip back to the mat.
8. Inhale as you lift up, exhale as you twist to face the mat, inhale as you face the ceiling, and exhale as you lower yourself back down.
9. Do two or three Twists on each side.

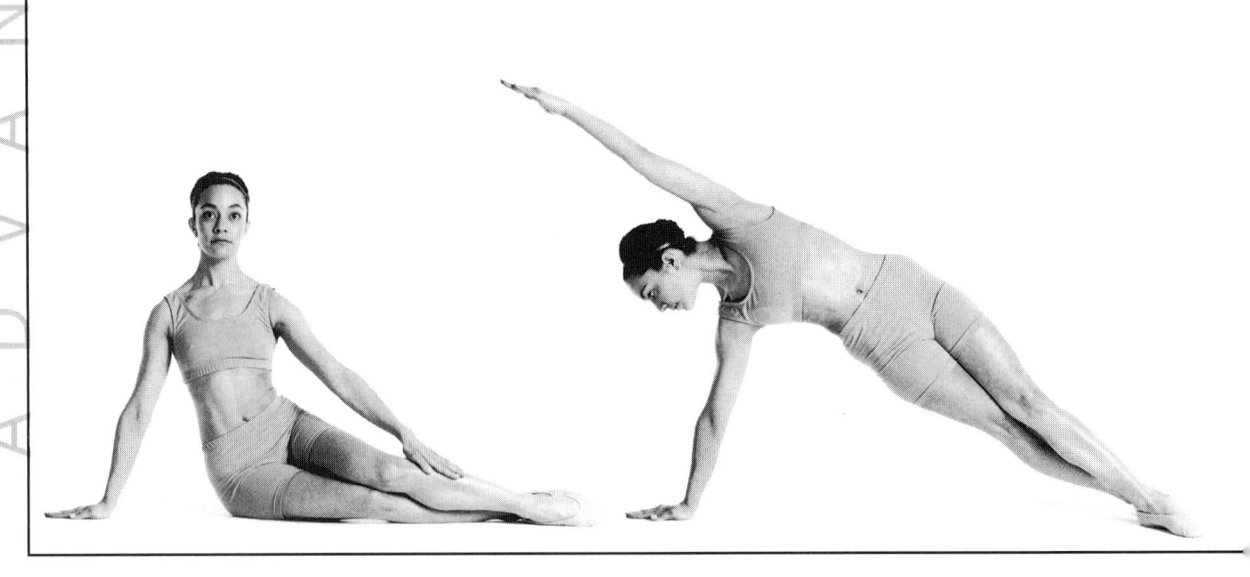

This extra puts your balance and control to the test. It works the major muscles of the abdominals, including your obliques, and stretches your hips and waistline.

The Extra Scoop

GOAL
- To maintain perfect balance and control in your hips while lengthening and twisting your upper body.

KEYS
- Stay reaching as long in your body as possible.
- Keep your hips still as you twist.
- Think of your feet being firmly planted as you perform the movements.

NO-NOS
- Do not let your hips or legs twist as you go.
- Do not sink into your shoulders or hips.
- Do not lean all your weight into your wrists or knees.

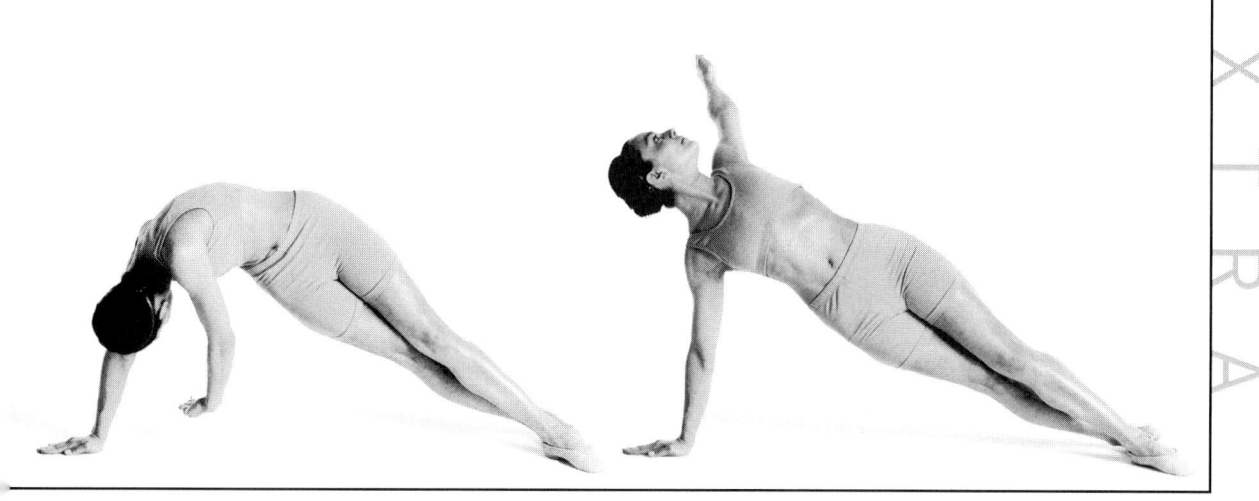

ADVANCED EXTRA

ROCKING

Step by Step

1. Lie on your stomach and bend your knees bringing your heels toward your bottom.
2. Reach behind you and grab your ankles (one at a time if necessary).
3. Inhaling, slowly stretch your body upward, lifting your chest and knees off the mat. Reach the soles of your feet to the back of your head. *Imagine you are being lifted to the ceiling by your hands and feet.*
4. Rock forward by pulling your ankles up toward your head and simultaneously pushing your chest to the mat. Exhale as you rock forward.
5. Inhale and rock back by lifting your chest and pulling back from your ankles. Keep your navel pressed to your spine. *Imagine yourself as a rocking horse.*
6. Rock back and forth five times. End by releasing your ankles and sitting back to your heels with your arms stretched long in front of you and your forehead on the mat. This will release the muscles of your lower back.

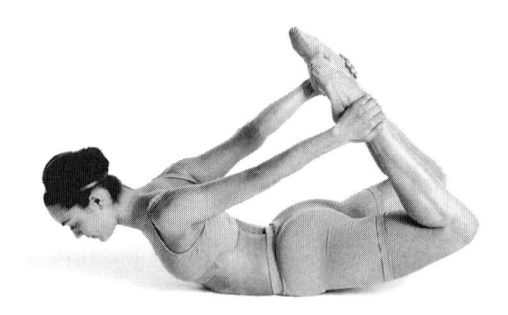

Rocking stretches your shoulders, back, quadriceps, and knees. It requires a strong back and a lot of abdominal control.

The Extra Scoop

GOAL
- To create a comfortable rhythm of breath and motion as you rock.

KEYS
- Use your breathing to provide the dynamic for the rocking.
- Keep your arms straight and your legs taut throughout.
- Constantly pull up in your chest and knees as you rock.
- Keep your head still and stretch your neck long to support the weight of your head.

NO-NOS
- Do not throw your head forward and back to initiate the rocking movements
- Do not allow your heels or hands to drop toward your bottom as you go.

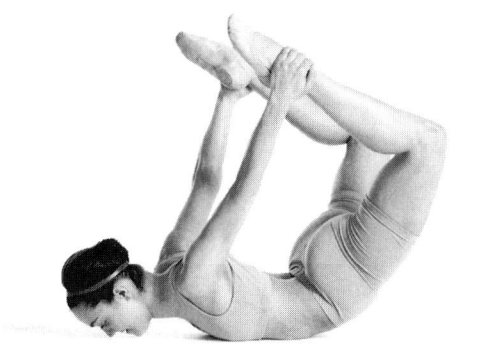

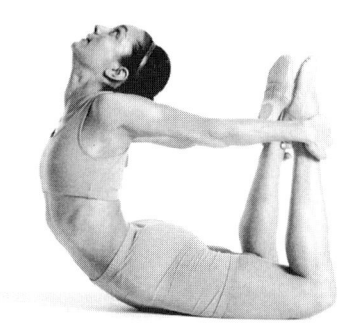

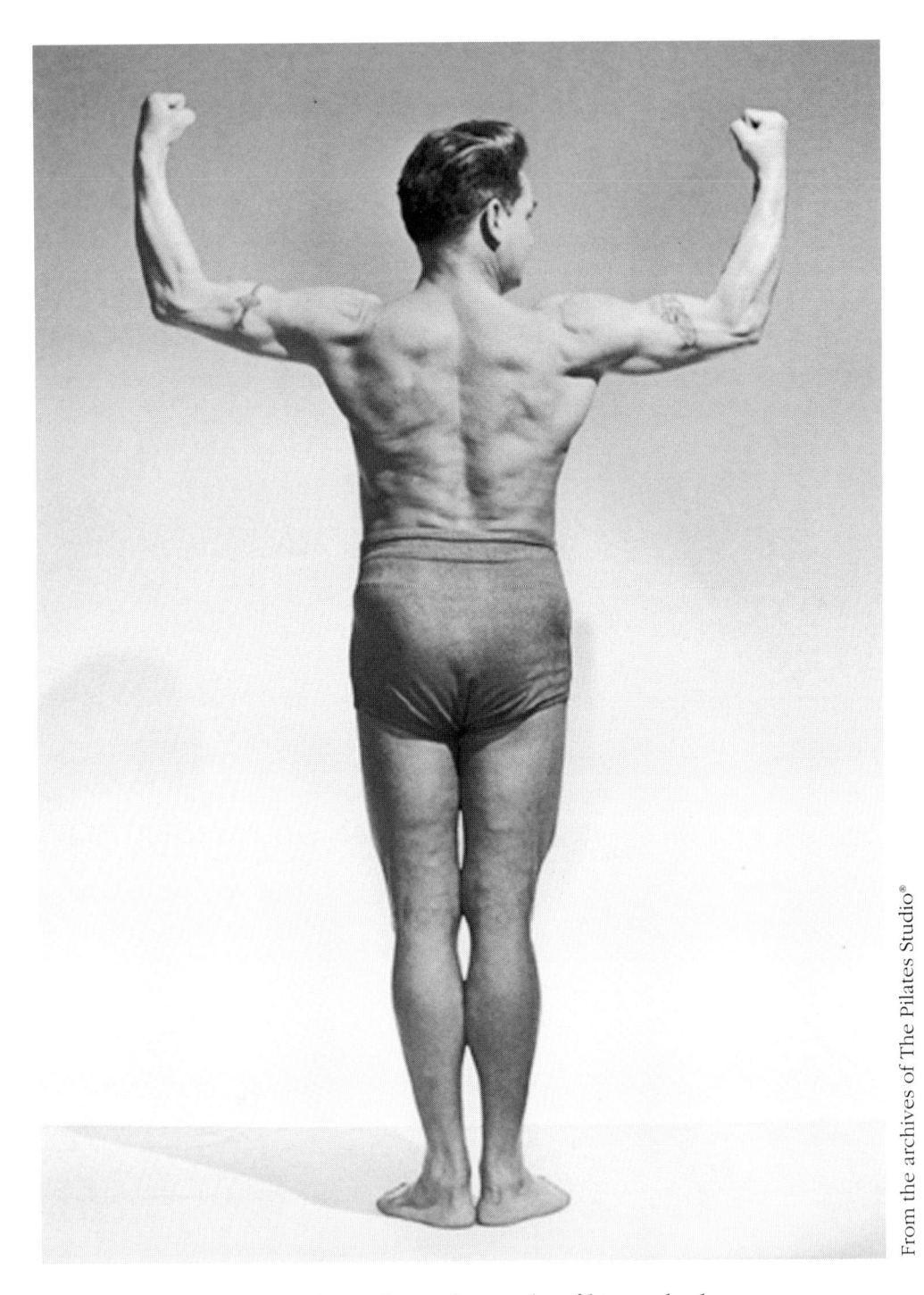

Joseph Pilates shows the results of his method.

The Standing Arm Series

1. Zip Up
2. Chest Expansion
3. Shaving the Head
4. Arm Circles
5. Biceps Curl I
6. Biceps Curl II
7. Triceps Extension
8. The Bug
9. Boxing
10. Lunges

These exercises can be performed with or without hand weights. (No more than two pounds is recommended.)

It is not necessary to perform all of the Standing Arm Series exercises each time. Choose the ones you feel best complement your workout level.

BEGINNER
ZIP UP

Step by Step

1. Stand in the Pilates stance with your arms hanging long in front of you.
2. Inhale and begin pulling your hands up the center line of your body, bending your elbows out to the sides as you go.
3. *Imagine you are pulling a tight zipper up your center line.*
4. Exhale and lower the hands and arms slowly, resisting gravity as you go.
5. *Imagine you are pressing down the heavy plunger on a box of dynamite.*
6. Do three to five sets, moving slowly and deliberately to create resistance.

- Rise up onto your toes as you "zip up" and lower your heels slowly as you press down.
- Do not allow your heels to come apart as you go.

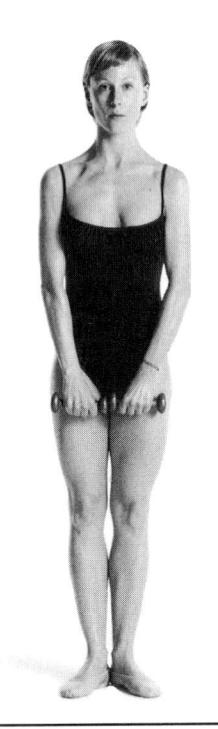

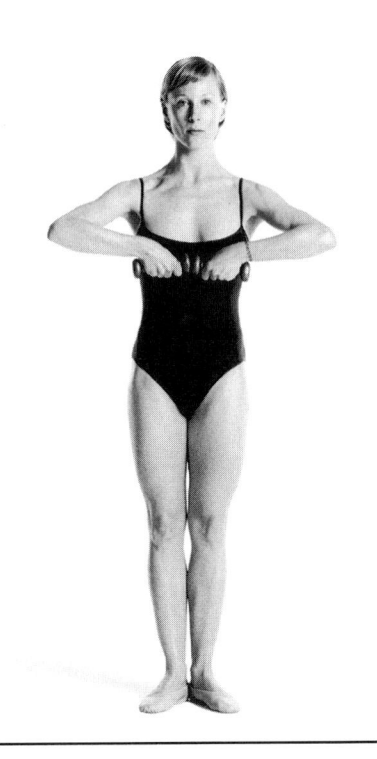

BEGINNER

CHEST EXPANSION

Step by Step

1. Stand in the Pilates stance with your arms long by your sides.
2. Inhale and press your palms back, lifting your chest open as you do.
3. Hold your breath as you turn your head slowly to the left and then to the right, stretching your neck and shoulder muscles. *Imagine pulling back on heavy springs attached to the wall in front of you.*
4. Return your head to center and exhale as you release your arms back down to your sides.
5. Repeat four sets, alternating the initial direction you turn your head each time.

- Rise onto your toes as you press your arms back and balance there as you turn your head from side to side. Lower your heels as you exhale and return to the starting position.

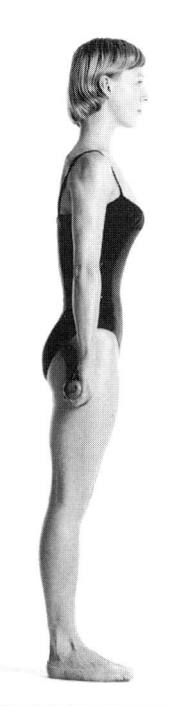

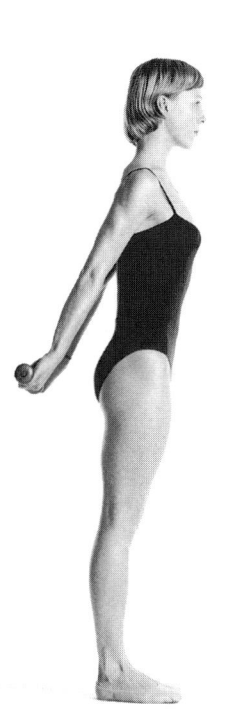

BEGINNER

SHAVING THE HEAD

Step by Step

1. Stand in the Pilates stance with your hands held in a triangle behind your head. Do not lift your shoulders as you perform the movements of this exercise.
2. Inhale and press your hands upward on a slight diagonal forward. *Imagine you are rolling a large boulder up a steep mountain with your hands.*
3. Exhale and slowly bring your hands back behind your head, *imagining the weight of the boulder hovering above your head as you do.*
4. Use your powerhouse to control your movements.
5. Repeat the sequence five times.

- Rise onto your toes as you stretch your arms up, and lower your heels as you exhale and return to your original position.
- Do not allow your heels to come apart as you go.

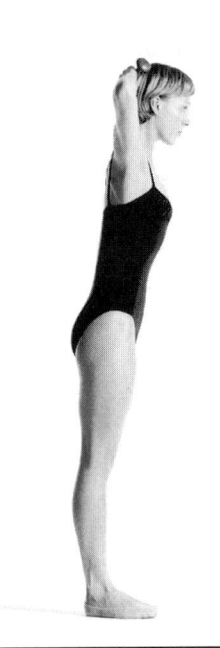

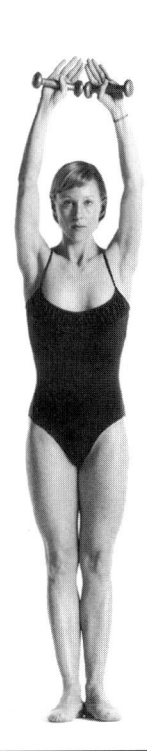

162

BEGINNER
ARM CIRCLES

Step by Step

1. Stand in the Pilates stance with your arms hanging long in front of you.
2. Begin making small, controlled circles with your arms as you raise them in front of you.
3. Make sure you are circling your entire arm from your shoulder and not from your wrist or forearm. *Imagine you are holding a heavy bucket in each hand.*
4. Continue circling until your arms are above your shoulders and then reverse the circles as you lower them back to your sides.
5. Make sure that your shoulders are pressing down and away from your ears as you perform the lifting and lowering motions.
6. Complete three to five sets of lifting and lowering your circling arms.

- Rise onto your toes as you circle your arms upward and then lower your heels back to the mat as you lower your arms.
- If you are performing the movements correctly, you should be able to feel your powerhouse working throughout the exercise. Remember to keep your body weight shifted slightly forward and over your toes.

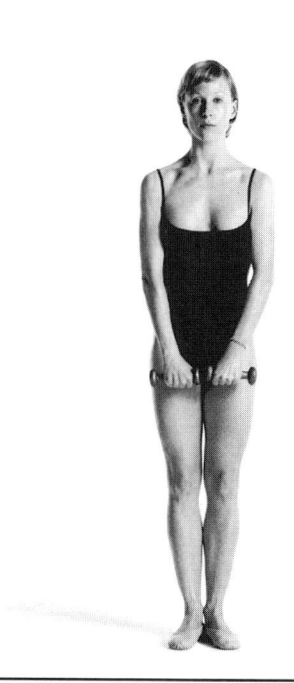

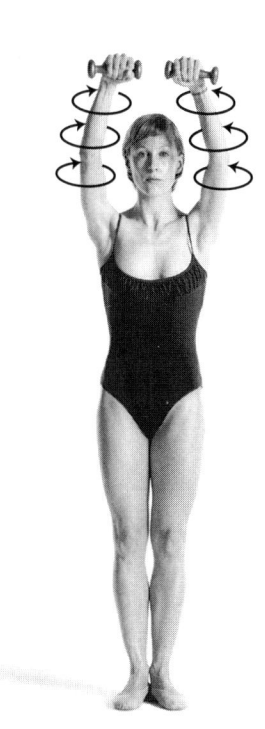

BEGINNER
BICEPS CURL I

Step by Step

1. Stand in the Pilates stance with your arms extended straight out in front of you, your hands made into fists with your palms facing the ceiling.
2. Inhale and slowly curl your wrists and forearms in toward your shoulders, *as if you were pulling on two heavy springs attached to the wall in front of you.*
3. Exhale and slowly uncurl your arms to their starting position, *trying to resist the pull of the imagined springs.*
4. Do not allow your elbows to drop as you perform the curling and uncurling movements.
5. Keep your shoulders pressing down and away from your ears.
6. Complete three to five repetitions.

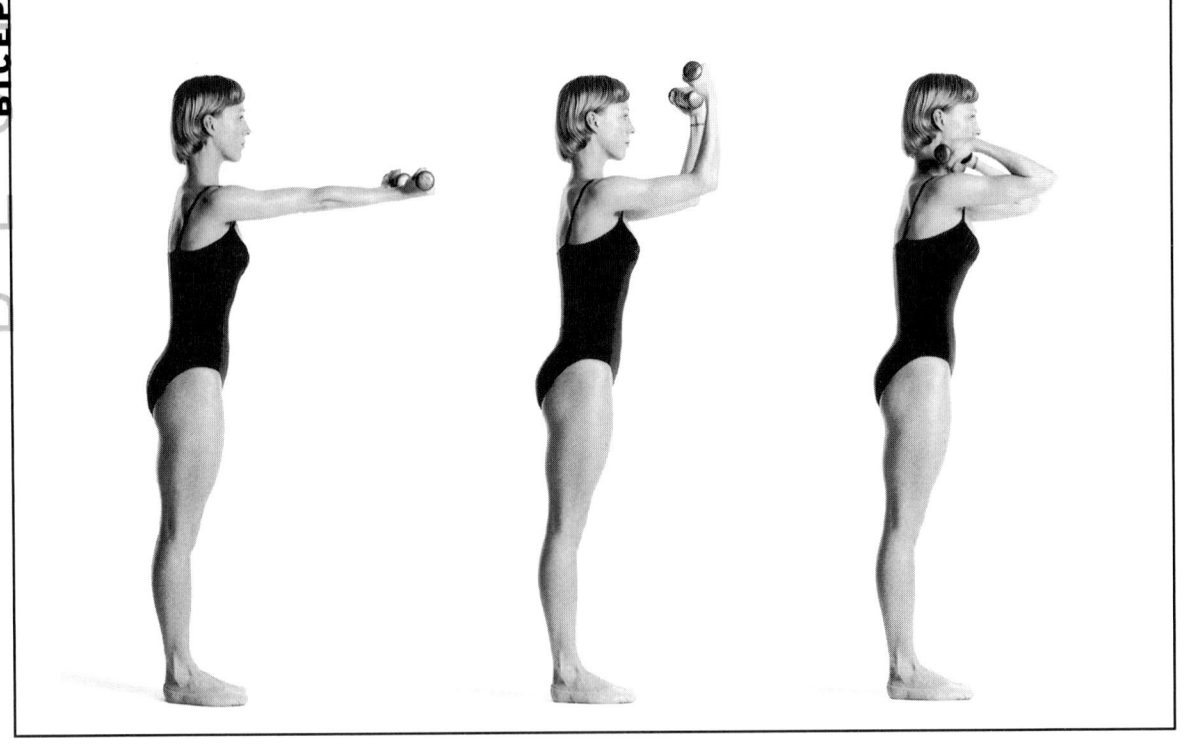

BEGINNER
BICEPS CURL II

Step by Step

1. Stand in the Pilates stance with your arms held out to your sides, hands made into fists with your palms facing the ceiling.
2. Make sure that your arms are slightly in front of your shoulders so that your hands are still within your peripheral vision.
3. Inhale, curling your wrists and forearms in toward your shoulders in a slow and controlled motion, *as if you were pulling on heavy pulleys attached to the walls.*
4. Exhale and *resist their pull* as you slowly uncurl your arms back to their starting position.
5. Do not allow your shoulders to lift as you curl your arms in.
6. Make sure that your elbows are aligned with your shoulders throughout the entire movement.
7. Complete three to five repetitions.

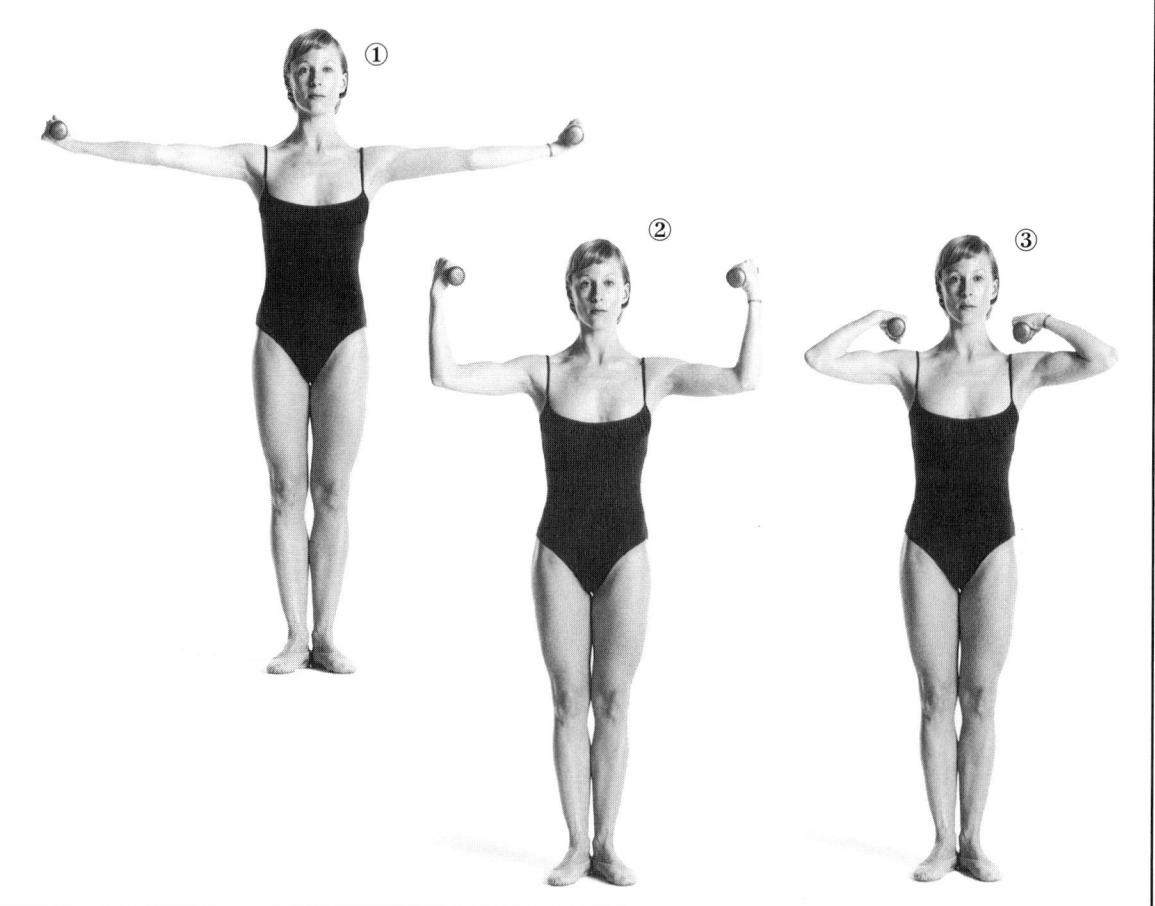

INTERMEDIATE
TRICEPS EXTENSION

Step by Step

1. Stand with your feet parallel and aligned directly beneath your hips.
2. Bend your knees deeply until your kneecaps are over your toes.
3. Fold your upper body forward until your back *is as straight as a tabletop,* and make sure that your head is aligned with your spine.
4. With your hands made into fists, palms facing each other, bend your elbows tightly into your sides and bring your fists to your shoulders.
5. Inhale and slowly extend your arms out straight behind you, *as if pulling on two springs attached to the wall in front of you.*
6. Make sure that you allow your arms to straighten fully without moving your elbows from their position tight against your sides.
7. Exhale and *resist the pull of the imagined springs* as you slowly bring your hands back into your shoulders.
8. Keep your knees bent and use your powerhouse to control your movements.
9. Complete three to five repetitions.

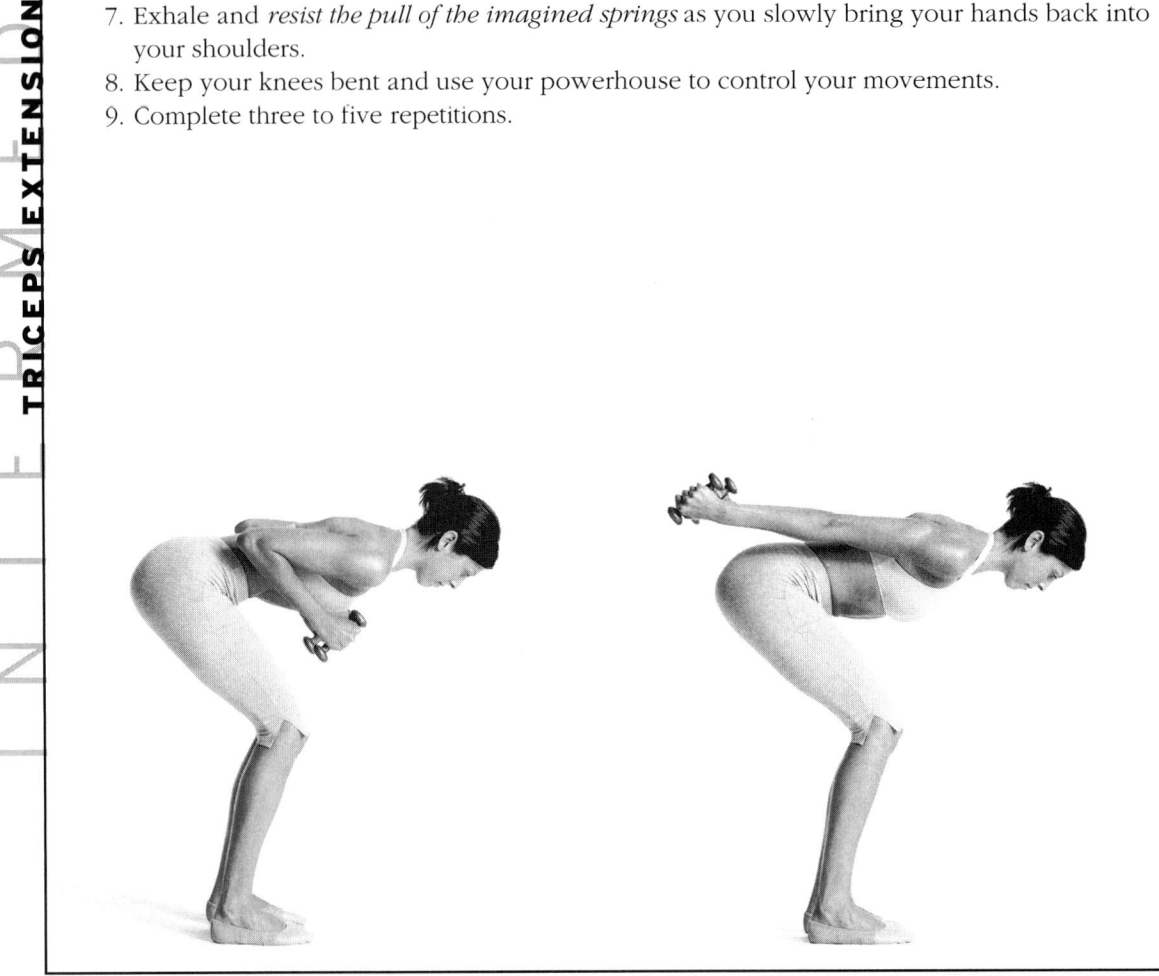

INTERMEDIATE

THE BUG

Step by Step

1. Stand with your feet parallel and aligned directly beneath your hips. *(Try to draw an imaginary line from your hip bones to the center of your heels.)*
2. Bend your knees deeply until your kneecaps are over your toes.
3. Fold your upper body forward until your back is straight and allow your arms to hang straight down toward the mat.
4. With your hands in fists and your knuckles facing each other, open your elbows out to either side.
5. In a slow and controlled motion, inhale and begin lifting your elbows up until they are aligned with your shoulders. *Imagine you are trying to open heavy trap doors*.
6. Exhale and *resist the pull of the doors* as you slowly bring your fists back togther.
7. Make sure that your head remains aligned with your spine and does not hang forward or lift back. *Imagine pressing the crown of your head into the wall in front of you.*
8. If your back hurts during this sequence, stop. Round forward and *roll* yourself back up to a standing position.
9. Remember to keep your knees bent and in alignment with your hips, and use your powerhouse to control the movements.
10. Complete three to five repetitions.

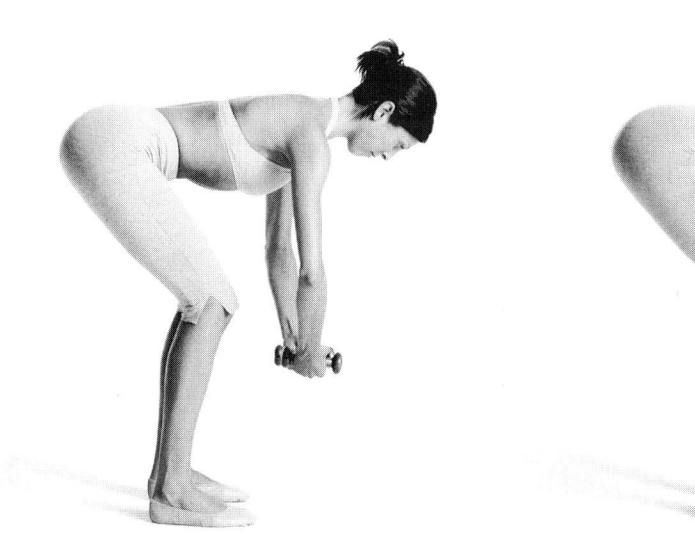

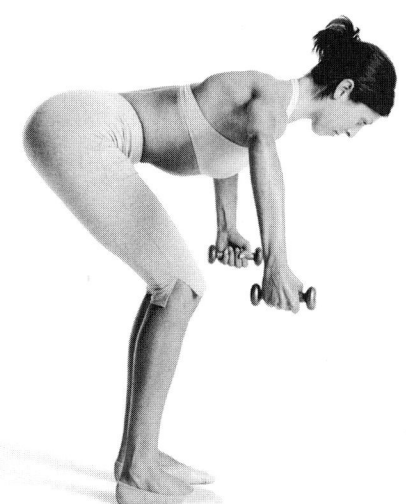

ADVANCED
BOXING

Step by Step

1. Take the starting position of the Triceps Extension (p. 166).
2. Inhale and simultaneously extend one arm straight out in front of you and one arm straight behind you. Turn your wrists as you perform this motion so that your front palm is facing down and your back palm is facing up.
3. Exhale and return your fists into your sides.
4. Inhale as you repeat the sequence with the opposite arm leading. Make sure that your extended arms are aligned with your body, neither lifted above nor dropping below.
5. Complete three to five sets.
- Do not throw your arms forward or back.
- This movement is slow and controlled, aligned from your powerhouse.

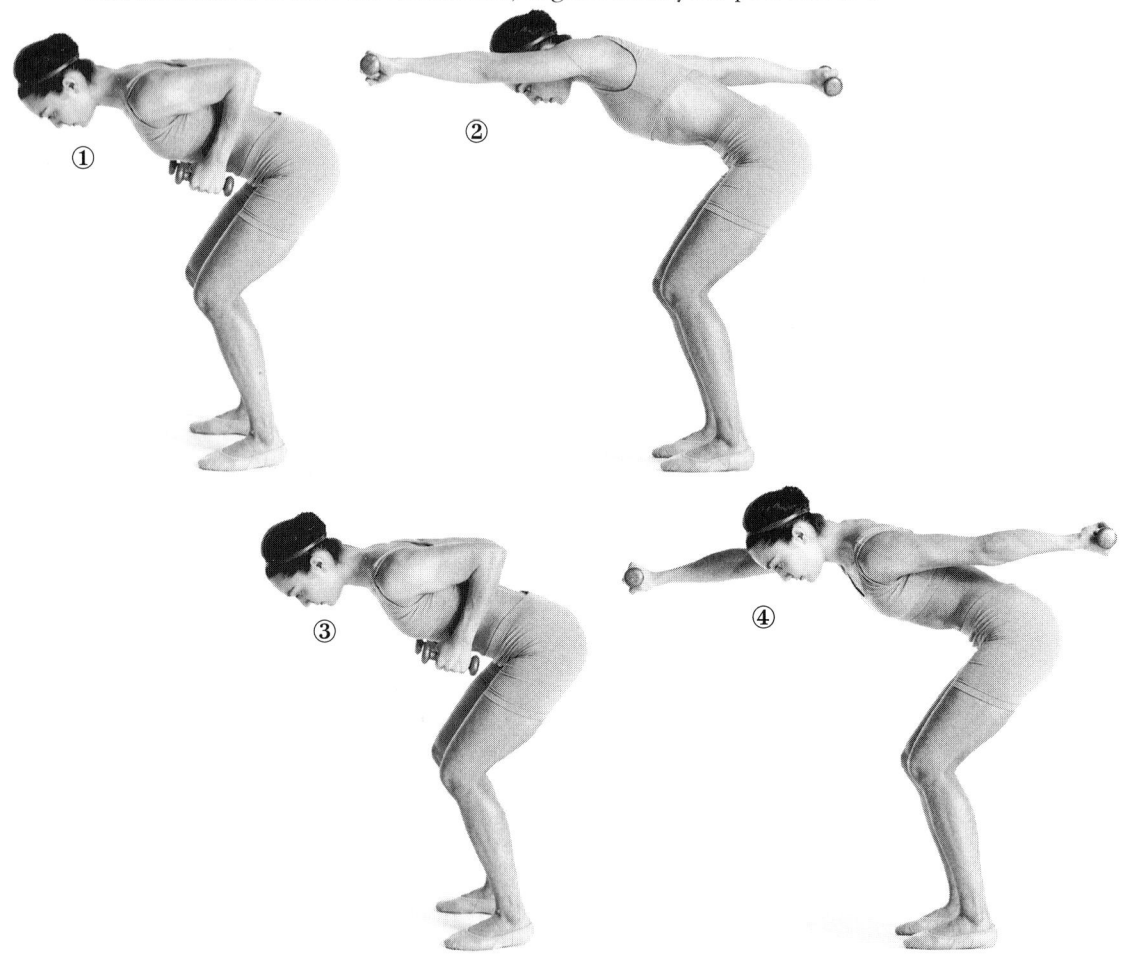

ADVANCED
LUNGES

Step by Step

1. Stand in a modified Pilates stance with the heel of your left foot against the arch of your right (third position in dance).
2. Twist your upper body to face left with your arms long by your sides.
3. In one swift and controlled motion, step your left foot out on a diagonal lunge and lean your upper body toward it, bringing your arms up alongside your ears. Inhale as you lunge. *Imagine holding back a crowd.*
4. Exhaling, push off your left foot and come back to your starting position.
5. Complete three lunges to each side.

- In the outstretched lunge position, lower and lift your straight arms without moving your torso. Keep the back of your neck long and the crown of your head stretching to the wall for stability. Exhale as you lower your arms, inhale as you lift them. Do no more than three repetitions.
- Do not lower your hips below your knee as you lunge.
- Keep your knee directly over your lunging foot for proper alignment.
- Do not rest your torso on your thigh when you lunge.
- Press back into your straight leg to evenly distribute your weight.
- Keep your navel pressed deeply into your spine throughout the movements.

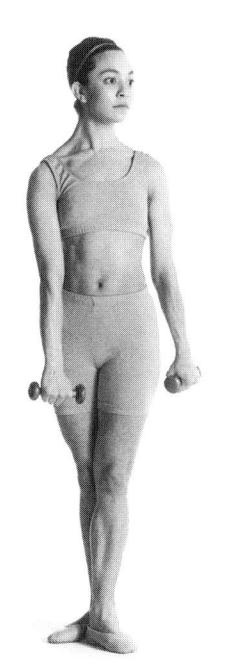

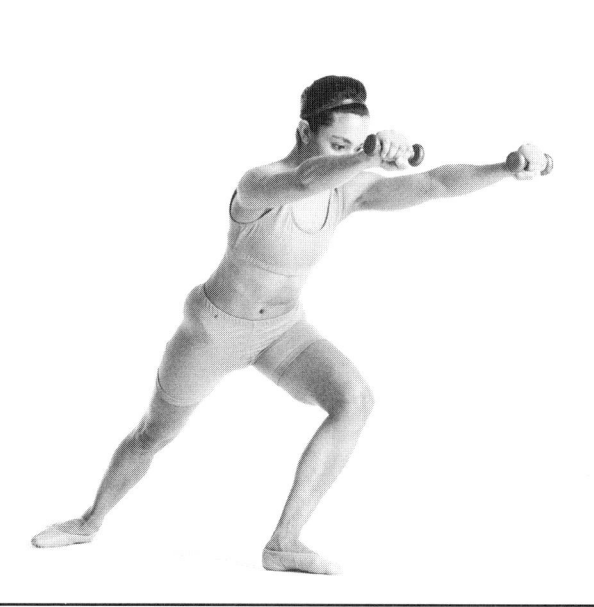

The Wall
(Cooldown)

1. Circles
2. Sliding Down
3. Rolling Down

CIRCLES ON THE WALL

Step by Step

1. Stand with your back against a wall and your feet about six to ten inches away from the base and in the Pilates stance.
2. Press your back flat so that all your vertebrae are touching the wall behind you.
3. Begin circling your arms in front of you, making sure not to lift them above shoulder height or to allow your hands out of your peripheral vision. *Imagine you are holding a heavy can of paint in each hand.*
4. Inhale as you begin the circle and exhale as you complete it.
5. Complete five circles in each direction.

The Inside Scoop

- Make sure that you do not arch your lower back away from the wall as you go.
- Keep your shoulders pressing down and away from your ears so that you are using the muscles of your powerhouse and not your shoulders to perform the circling motion.
- You may find it difficult in the beginning to get your entire spine flat, so make sure that at least your mid- and lower back make contact with the wall.
- Keep lifting taller as you go. Do not allow yourself to sink into your lower back or shoulders.

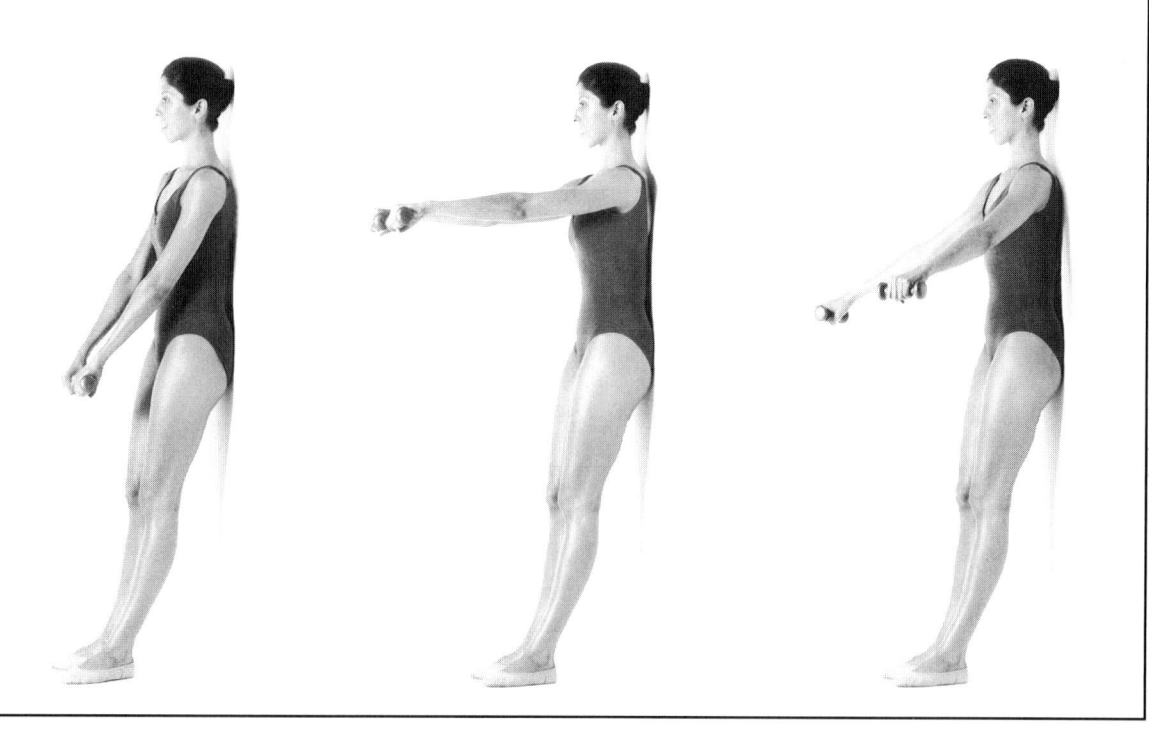

SLIDING DOWN THE WALL

Step by Step

1. Standing with your back pressed up against the wall, position your feet so that they are hip's width apart and about six to eight inches out from the wall. (This will vary depending on your height.)
2. Begin sliding your back down the wall by bending your knees. Keep your knees aligned with your hips and do not allow yourself to slide down so far that your bottom is below the height of your knees. Stop when you feel you can comfortably maintain a seated position.
3. Make sure that your entire spine maintains contact with the wall behind you by continuing to work from your powerhouse. *Imagine you are being pulled back by a powerful magnet behind the wall*.
4. Inhale as you slide down and then hold your breath as long as possible.
5. Exhale and slide yourself back up the wall by pressing into the soles of your feet.
6. Repeat the sequence three times, holding the down position as long as possible.

- In the seated position you can add the arm circles from page 163, or simply raise your arms to shoulder height as you slide down and lower your arms as you slide up as in the photos below. Hold your arms at shoulder height as you hold your breath. Exhale as you lower them.

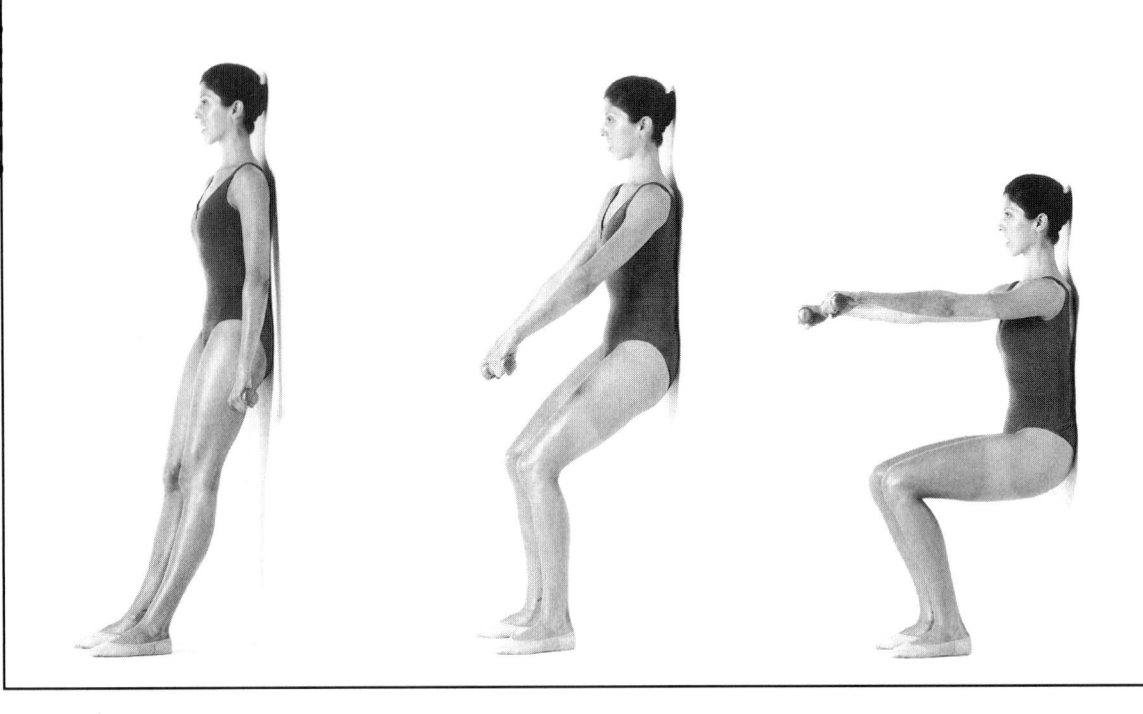

ROLLING DOWN THE WALL

Do this exercise whenever you need to relax, or at the end of a workout to stretch your muscles.

Step by Step

1. Stand with your back pressed flat against a wall and your feet in the Pilates stance about eight to ten inches from the base of the wall.
2. Inhale and begin rolling down by bringing your chin to your chest and then "peeling" each vertebra from the wall. Imagine rubber cement sticking you to the wall as you roll down.
3. Roll down only to the point where your tailbone still maintains contact with the wall behind you, and allow your arms to hang loosely as you go.
4. Pull your navel deeply into your spine to increase the stretch. Engage all the muscles of your powerhouse to maintain control in this position. Imagine you are leaning over a railing.
5. Allow your arms to circle freely and relax your head and neck. Breathe naturally.
6. After five circles in each direction inhale and roll back up the wall, replacing each vertebra as you go.

The Inside Scoop

- Use your powerhouse and not your head to come up. (Your head should be the last part to lift up.)
- You may find that you need to soften your knees or slightly tuck your pelvis to begin rolling up.
- Make sure that you end by pressing your entire spine back into the wall, opening your chest and exhaling.

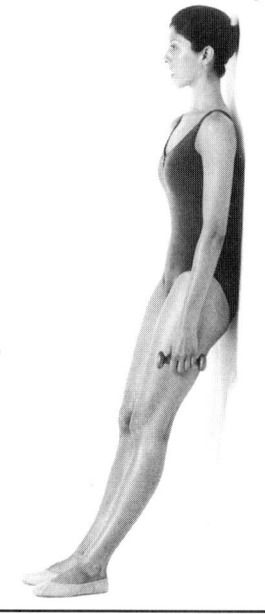

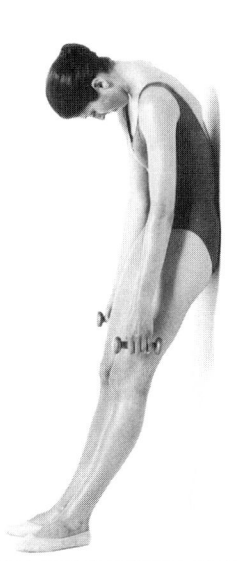

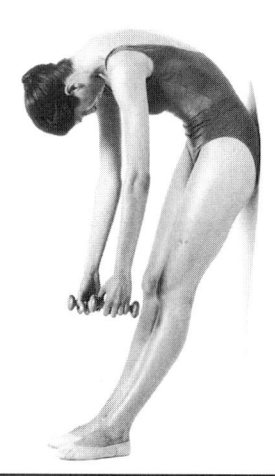

The Next Step

If you are looking to work with a certified Pilates instructor, here is a list of teachers around the world. For the most up-to-date information, please visit www.pilates-studio.com.

The Pilates Studio® Certifying Centers
© Copyright 1999 Pilates Inc., Pilates® and the Pilates Studio®
are registered trademarks of Pilates Inc. www.pilates-studio.com

NEW YORK CITY *(West Side)*	The Pilates Studio®, Sean P. Gallagher, PT, Director, 2121 Broadway, Suite 201, New York, NY 10023 (between 74th and 75th Sts.), (212) 875-0189, Fax: (212) 769-2368, Purchase Products: (888) 278-7227 x23
(Midtown)	Drago's Gym, Romana Kryzanowska, Sari Pace, Master Teacher, 50 West 57th St., 6th Fl., New York, NY 10019, (212) 757-0724
FLORIDA *Fort Myers*	The Pilates Studio® of Fort Myers, Hope Petrine, Director/Certified Instructor, 11751 Cleveland Ave., Suites 21 and 22, Fort Myers, FL 33907, (941) 274-5711, Fax: (941) 274-6622
ILLINOIS *Evanston*	The Pilates Studio® of the Midwest, Fatima Bruhns, Director/Instructor, 820 Davis St., Suite 202, Evanston, IL 60201, (847) 492-0464, Fax: (847) 492-0210
WASHINGTON *Seattle*	The Pilates Studio® of Seattle & Capitol Hill Physical Therapy, Lauren Stephen, Lori Coleman Brown, PT, Directors/Instructors, 413 Fairview Ave. North, Seattle, WA 98109, (206) 405-3560, Fax: (206) 405-3938
PENNSYLVANIA *Philadelphia*	The Pilates Studio® @ the P.A. Ballet, June Hines, Megan Egan, Instructors, 1101 South Broad St., Philadelphia, PA 19147, (215) 551-7000, Fax: (215) 551-7224
GEORGIA *Atlanta*	The Pilates Studio® @ the Atlanta Ballet, Denise Reeves, Director/Instructor, 4279 Roswell Rd., #703, Atlanta, GA 30342, (404) 459-9555, Fax: (404) 459-9455
BRAZIL *São Paulo*	The Pilates Studio®, Inelia Garcia, Director/Instructor: R. Estevan, Cecilia Delgado. R. Cincinato Braga, Instructors, 520 Bela Vista, São Paulo, Brazil, Tel./Fax: 011-55112848905
AUSTRALIA *Surry Hills*	The New York Studio of Pilates® of Australia, Cynthia Lochard, Director/Instructor, Roula Karitarzoglou, Edwina Ward, Instructors, Suite 12, Level 4146-56 Holt St., Surry Hills, 2010 Australia, Tel./Fax: 011-61296984689

Instructors Certified by the Pilates Studio®

ALABAMA
Gulf Shores — Misti McKee, Instructor, Gulf Shores, AL 36542, (334) 955-6466

ALASKA
Fairbanks — Ann Turner, Instructor, 621 Gingko Rd., Fairbanks, AK 99709, (907) 479-2360

ARIZONA
Phoenix — Fitness Solutions, Inc., Lauren Tomasulo, Owner/Instructor, 4515 North 16th St., Suite 113, Phoenix, AZ 85016, (602) 631-9698

Phoenix — Pamela More, Instructor, Tel./Fax: (602) 569-1612

Phoenix — Pamela LaPierre, Phoenix, AZ 85008, (602) 817-4402

Scottsdale — Studio Joe, Joey Greco, Sherry Brady Greco, Janice Wessman, Pratibha Noggle, Instructors, 7170 East McDonald, #5, Scottsdale, AZ 85253, (602) 367-8501

Scottsdale — Harry Zabrocki, Alicia Elliott, Instructors, (602) 538-3046

Scottsdale — Janice Wessman, Instructor, Tel./Fax: (602) 675-8501, wessmanj@aol.com

Tucson — John White, Instructor, 2025 North Nancy Rose Blvd., Tucson, AZ 85712, (520) 319-8242

Tucson — Jennifer Pollack, Instructor, Tucson, AZ 85719, (520) 320-7844

Tucson — Suzanne Rosin, Jerome Weinberg, Instructors, 7001 Eagle Point Pl., Tucson, AZ 85750, (520) 299-0544

Tucson — Debi Crawford, Instructor, 5451 North Via Del Arbolito, Tucson, AZ 85750, (520) 577-1597, dlcrawf@aol.com

CALIFORNIA
Alhambra — Powerhouse, Sasha Koziak, Instructor, 1003 Bushnell St., Alhambra, CA 91801, (526) 458-5600, jkoziak@earthlink.net

Berkeley — Minoo Hamzavi, Instructor, 1525 Spruce St., #36, Berkeley, CA 94709-1561, (510) 848-4133

Berkeley — Mirta Lee Ribas, Instructor, 1315 Stannage Ave., Berkeley, CA 94702, (510) 558-9010, birthrites@igc.org

Brentwood — Above and Beyond Fitness, Sara Carone, Instructor, 11601 Wilshire Blvd., Brentwood, CA 90049, (310) 966-1999

Burbank — Regina Fox Dawson, Instructor, (818) 559-3509, regdawson@yahoo.com

Burbank — Merilee Blaisdell, Instructor, (818) 504-9630, MerileeMB@aol.com

Calabasas Hills — Jacqueline Berns, Instructor, (310) 317-0990

Encino — Michael Levy Workout, Michael Levy, Linda Luber, Karen Biancardi, Sarah Lovatt Carone, Instructors, 17200 Ventura Blvd., #310, Encino, CA 91316, (818) 783-0097

Glendale — The Gold Touch, Darien Gold, Owner/Instructor, 610 North Jackson St., Glendale, CA 91206, (888) 908-4778

For the most up-to-date information, please visit www.pilates-studio.com.

Hollywood	Bill and Jacqui Landrum, Instructors, 6315 Ivarene Ave., Hollywood, CA 90068, (323) 469-2012
Irvine	Audrey Wilson, Instructor, 30 Seton Rd., Irvine, CA 92715, (949) 551-3443, audreydancin@earthlink.net
Lomita/Torrance	Joellyn Musser, Instructor, 24725 Pennsylvania Ave., C-19, Lomita, CA 90717, (310) 530-7881, clbr8lkif@earthlink.net
Los Angeles	Licia Perea, Instructor, 2159 Lyric Ave., Los Angeles, CA 90027, (323) 669-3303
Los Angeles	Jennifer Palmer, Instructor, (323) 394-5469
Los Angeles	Niedra Gabriel (known formerly as Mickey Terra), Karen Biancardi, Instructors, 616 North Spaulding Ave., Los Angeles, CA 90036, (323) 651-1796
Los Angeles	Charlene Hanson, Instructor, 1745 Beloit Ave., #117, Los Angeles, CA 90025, (310) 312-8942
Los Angeles	Renda Mishalany, Instructor, $332^{1}/_{2}$ North Orange Grove Ave., Los Angeles, CA 90036, (213) 525-0293
Los Angeles	Laurel Canyon Studio, Heidi Kling, Instructor, 8549 Walnut Dr., Los Angeles, CA 90046, (323) 654-4347, Fax: (323) 654-2396
Los Angeles	Karen Biancardi, 571 N. Gower, Los Angeles, CA 90004, (213) 957-2035
Los Angeles	Geoffrey Rhue, Instructor, 2127 Yosemite Dr., Los Angeles, CA 90041, (213) 254-8490
Los Angeles	Nonna Glazer, Instructor, 310 South Hamel, #103, Los Angeles, CA 90048, (310) 385-9485
Malibu	Survival of the Fittest, Jacqueline Berns, Instructor, 3806-J Cross Creek Rd., Malibu, CA 90265, (310) 317-0990
Malibu	Phyllis Reffo, Instructor, 30125 Harvester Rd., Malibu, CA 90265, (310) 457-8751
Newport Beach	Body Fit, Sheena Jongeneel, Instructor, 3422 Via Lido, Newport Beach, CA 92663, (949) 675-2639
North Hills	Sarah Lovatt-Carone, Instructor, 9219 Hagvenhurst Ave., North Hills, CA 91344, (818) 893-5387
North Hollywood	Trish Garland Studio, Trish Garland, Instructor, 12223 Califa St., North Hollywood, CA 91607, (818) 985-8222
Oakland	Katherine Davis, Instructor, Oakland, CA 94610, (510) 832-0653, KDavis5267@aol.com
Oceanside (San Diego Area)	Julia Hilleary, Instructor, Oceanside, CA 92056, (760) 431-7988
Ojai	Mary Jo Healy, Jinny Feiss, Instructors, 218 North Padre Juan Ave., Ojai, CA 93023, (805) 646-3797, Fax: (805) 640-8930, healy@ojai.net
Pasadena	ZOE, Zoe Hagler, Owner/Instructor/Teacher/Trainer, Geoffrey Rhue, Merilee Blaisdell, Jennifer Palmer, Instructors, 21 South El Molino, Pasadena, CA 91101, (626) 585-8853

For the most up-to-date information, please visit www.pilates-studio.com.

Redondo Beach	Arlene Renay Reese, Instructor, 313 Avenue G, Redondo Beach, CA 90277, (310) 540-5539
San Diego	Studio Mo, Moses Urbano, Instructor, (619) 295-1850, Fax: (619) 295-1023, studiomo@home.com
San Francisco	Catherine Kirsch, Instructor, (415) 288-1001 x7064, Cherrie_34@hotmail.com
San Francisco	Kerri Palmer Gonon, Instructor, San Francisco, CA 94131, (415) 441-6985, twoinsf@flash.net or kp_trainer@yahoo.com
San Francisco	Nancy Rosellini, Instructor, 387 Staples Ave., San Francisco, CA 94112, (415) 441-6985
Santa Monica	Nela Fry, Instructor, 1008 Euclid St., Santa Monica, CA 90403, Tel./Fax: (310) 394-2805, nela@csi.com
Santa Monica	Heather Leon, Instructor, 508A Santa Monica Blvd, Santa Monica, CA 90401, (310) 394-9780
Santa Monica	Jennifer Bocian, Instructor, (310) 260-9736
Santa Monica	Unda Joy Luber, 932 17th Pl., Santa Monica, CA 90403, (310) 588-7376
Sherman Oaks	The Body Coach, Susan Lonergan, Instructor, (818) 905-6856
Sherman Oaks	Courtney, Instructor, (818) 986-8361
West Hollywood	Winsor Fitness, Mari Winsor, Instructor, 945 North LaCienega, West Hollywood, CA 90069, (310) 289-8766, Fax: (310) 289-0812
Westlake Village	Deborah Mandis Cozen, RPT, Instructor, 3034 Winding Lane, Westlake Village, CA 91361, (805) 373-1030
Westwood	Adylia Roman, Instructor, Westwood, CA 90024, (310) 446-6100

COLORADO

Boulder	Flatiron Athletic Club, Deidre Szarabajka, Michelle Perkins, Instructors, 505 Thunderbird Dr., Boulder, CO 80301, (303) 499-6590, www.FACBoulder.com
Breckenridge	Jessica Paffrath, Instructor, Breckenridge, CO 80424, (970) 453-2139
Denver	Amy Halaby, Instructor (Denver Athletic Club), 1325 Glenarm Pl., Denver, CO 80204, (303) 534-7331 x1502

CONNECTICUT

Bridgeport	Monica Mauri, Instructor, Bridgeport, CT 06605, (203) 333-8926
Cos Cob	Terese Garsson, Instructor, 14 Pond Pl., Cos Cob, CT 06807 (near Greenwich and Stamford), (203) 629-5543, Tgarsson@aol.com
Greenwich	The Fitness Edge, Mejo Wiggin, Saro Vanasup, Caroline Benton, Instructors, (203) 629-3743
Greenwich	Patricia Erickson, Instructor, P.O. Box 7737, Greenwich, CT 06836, Tel./Fax: (203) 661-1848, pattyerick@aol.com
New Canaan	Holly Mensching, Instructor, 11 Burtis Ave., New Canaan, CT 06840, (203) 972-3438

For the most up-to-date information, please visit www.pilates-studio.com.

New Haven	Lenore Frost, CHT, OTR/L, Instructor, 61 Amity Rd., Suite B, New Haven, CT 06515, (203) 389-8177
Norfolk	Sarah Smolen, Instructor, (860) 542-0081
Norwalk	Oleg Belousou, Instructor, (203) 847-0591
Ridgefield	Simone Wunderli-Rucolas, Instructor, 124 Tanton Hill Rd., Ridgefield, CT 06877, (203) 438-7984, Swisssimi@aol.com
South Norwalk	Amy Matton, Instructor, South Norwalk, CT 06854, (203) 831-8701
Thomaston	Jeffrey Smolen, Instructor, (860) 283-6428
West Hartford	Elizabeth Flores, Instructor, 41 South Main St., West Hartford, CT 06107, (860) 233-5232
Westport	Bodywork Studio, Cristina Bruno, Lynn Bartner, Ossi Rauch, Jeanne Turkel, Instructors, 645 Post Rd. East, Westport, CT 06880, (203) 226-8550, Fax: (203) 222-0731
Westport	Lynn Bartner, Instructor, LMB21665@aol.com

FLORIDA

Boca Raton	The Balanced Body Inc., Cecil S. Y. Ybanez, PT, Instructor, 5580 North Federal Hwy., Boca Raton, FL 33487, (561) 994-8848
Boca Raton	Boca Body Works, Cindy Maybruck, Instructor, 7088 Beracasa Way, Boca Raton, FL 33433, (561) 347-1110, Fax: (561) 395-7544, cmaybruck@aol.com
Burnell	Robin Campbell, Instructor, (904) 437-6022
Delray Beach	John Mahoney, Instructor, 39 Gleason St., Delray Beach, FL 33483, (561) 703-5646
Fort Lauderdale	Martha (Marty) Hammerstein, 516 Southwest 12th Ct., Fort Lauderdale, FL 33315, (954) 525-8565
Fort Myers	The Pilates Studio® of Fort Myers, Hope Petrine, Director/Certified Instructor, 11751 Cleveland Ave., Suites 21 and 22, Fort Myers, FL 33907, (941) 274-5711, Fax: (941) 2746622
Miami	Progressive Bodyworks of Miami, Anna Caban, Instructor, 3622 Northeast 2nd Ave., Miami, FL 33137, (305) 438-0555, Fax: (305) 438-0545, www.pro-body.com
Miami Beach	Alba Calzada Carter, Instructor, 1674 Meridian Ave., #506, Miami Beach, FL 33139, (305) 695-8084
Orlando	Mod Bod 2000, Jacki Garland, Jessica Gazzola, Samantha Gazzda, Instructors, (407) 903-0641
St. Petersburg	Linda McNamar, Instructor, 1045 9th Ave. North, St. Petersburg, FL 33705, (727) 822-4722
Sarasota	Dynamic Fitness Inc., Sherry Resh, Instructor, 4141 South Tamiami Trail, Suite 11, Sarasota, FL 34231, (941) 379-8811, S.Resh@aol.com
Winter Park	Michelle Hartog, Instructor, 4355 Bear Gully Rd., Winter Park, FL 32792, (407) 678-3116, mglowhart@aol.com

Winter Park	MatWorkz, Debra Watson, Instructor, 558 West New England Ave., #200, Winter Park, FL 32789, (407) 628-4888
GEORGIA	
Atlanta	The Pilates Studio® @ the Atlanta Ballet, Denise Reeves, Director/Instructor, Robin Warden, Deidra Simon, Emily Bradley, Cristina Williams, Instructors, 4279 Roswell Rd., #703, Atlanta, GA 30342, (404) 459-9555, Fax: (404) 459-9455
Atlanta	Studio Lotus, Misti McKee, Flo Fitzgerald, Instructors, 1123 Zonolite Rd., Suite 19, Atlanta, GA 30306, (404) 817-0900, www.studiolotus.com
Atlanta	Lisa Browning, Instructor, 3200 Cobb-Galeria Pkwy., #215, Atlanta, GA 30339, (770) 984-8889, LBSMT@aol.com
Duluth	Elizabeth Elliott, Instructor, (770) 623-3119, Lelliott2@aol.com
Norcross	The Work, Edgar Tirado, Instructor, 5952 Peachtree Ind. Blvd., #16, Norcross, GA, (770) 518-9610
HAWAII	
Pukalani	Belkis Lodzada, Instructor, Pukalani, HI 96788, (808) 572-7683
IDAHO	
Boise	Carrie Shanafelt, Instructor, (208) 345-6526
ILLINOIS	
Antioch	Patricia Kendziora, Instructor, (847) 395-2686
Barrington	Welcome to Your Body, Inc., Maryanne Radzis, Susan Hacker, Instructors, 220 South Cook St., Barrington, IL 60010, (847) 304-4900
Barrington	Susan Hacker, Instructor, (773) 489-9844
Chicago	Stacy Weitzner, Instructor, (773) 529-7104
Chicago	Juanita Lopez, Instructor/Teacher/Trainer, (312) 878-3639
Chicago	Julie Schiller, Instructor, 1016 North Dearborn, Chicago, IL 60610, (773) 871-2385
Chicago	Integrations, Inc., Kevin Bradley, Instructor, 1122 North Clark St., Chicago, IL 60610, (312) 280-7950
Chicago	David Englund, Instructor, 1912 Lincoln Park West, Chicago, IL 60714, (312) 932-0991, Mrerolfu@aol.com
Chicago	Chiropractic Health Resources, Corrine Stamslaw, Ceci Fano-Bryan, Jacqueline Brenner, Instructors, 2105 North Southport, #208, Chicago, IL 60614, (773) 472-0560
Chicago	Body Endeavors-Performance Gym, Liv Berger, Instructor, 1000 West North Ave., 3rd Fl., Chicago, IL 60622, (312) 202-0028, Fax: (312) 751-8122
Chicago	Gail Tangeros, Instructor, 1720 West Leland, #2, Chicago, IL 60640, (773) 561-2854
Chicago	Krista Merrill, Instructor, 5030 North Parkside Ave., Chicago, IL 60630, (773) 545-6165
Chicago	Susan Hacker, Instructor, (773) 489-9844

For the most up-to-date information, please visit www.pilates-studio.com.

Chicago	Fitness Foundations Chicago, Linda Tremain, PT, Krista Merrill, Juliet Cella, Instructors, 213 West Institute Pl., #303, Chicago, IL 60610, (312) 642-5633, Fax: (312) 642-5733, ltremain@sprynet.com
Chicago	Erin Harper, Instructor, 5313 North Ravenswood, #301, Chicago, IL 60640, (773) 989-9979
Chicago	The Pilates Studio® of the Midwest at Hubbard Dance Complex, Dana Santi, Manager, 1151 West Jackson Ave., Chicago, IL 60607, (312) 492-8835, Fax: (312) 492-8875
Chicago	The Pilates Studio® of the Midwest at Ballet Chicago, 185 North Wabash, Chicago, IL 60601
Chicago	Joe Palla, Instructor, 5828 North Paulina, Chicago, IL 60660, (773) 344-6491
Evanston	The Pilates Studio® of the Midwest, Fatima Bruhns, Director/Instructor, Juanita Lopez, Teacher of Teachers and Training Director, Loribeth Cohen, PT (Dir. of P.T.), Dorota Gottfried, Jenna Sisk, Rhonda Celenza, Dana Santi, Joe Palla, Ellen Krafft, Randi Neebe, Mary Nardi, Gail Tangeros, Gail Diehl, Instructors, 820 Davis St., Suite 202, Evanston, IL 60201, (847) 492-0464, Fax: (847) 492-0210
Glen Carbon	The Integrated Body, Pam Moody, Instructor, 23-C Kettle River Dr., Glen Carbon, IL 62034 (St. Louis Area), (618) 656-3890
Glenview	Loribeth Cohen, Instructor, 3122 Crestwood Lane, Glenview, IL 60025, (847) 998-5859 or (847) 624-7455
Highland Park	In Synch Fitness Corp., Fatima Bruhns, Director/Instructor, Debbie LaMantia, Randi Neebe, Joe Palla, Patty Kendziora, Instructors, 1898 First St., Highland Park, IL 60035, (847) 266-1512
Lake Villa	Cathie Deref-McCue, Instructor, 38569 Route 59, Lake Villa, IL 60046 (near border of WI), (847) 356-0180, CDM_HEALTHY_BODY@Juno.com
North Shore	Cheryl Ivey, Instructor, (847) 651-5413
Oakbrook	Fitness Foundations, Inc., Linda Tremain, PT, Jill Popovich, Amy McDowell, Krista Merrill, Erin Harper, Instructors, 1111 West 22nd St., #610, Oakbrook, IL 60523, (630) 573-5877, Fax: (630) 573-5875, ltremain@sprynet.com
Oak Park	Alternative Fitness Studio, Andrea Andrade, Instructor, 126 North Oak Park Ave., Oak Park, IL 60302, (708) 386-4930
Skokie	Barbara Stoltz, Instructor, 8700 Ridge Way, Skokie, IL 60076, (847) 677-3194
Willowbrook	Dana Santi, Instructor, 6141 Knoll Wood Rd., Willowbrook, IL 60514, (630) 654-9834, DanaST919@aol.com

IOWA
Bettendorf	Gail Diehl, Instructor, 4640 Crow Creek Ct., Bettendorf, IA 52722-6925, (319) 332-8625

KANSAS
Overland Park	Modern Body Contrology, David Mooney, Instructor, 9308 Dearborn, Overland Park, KS 66207, Tel./Fax: (913) 649-1479

LOUISIANA

New Orleans	Larry Gibas. Instructor, 1702 Fern St., New Orleans, LA 70118, (504) 862-6210
New Orleans	Monica Wilson, Instructor, (504) 894-1665, bwilson@mailhost.tes.tulane.edu
New Orleans	Caroline Probst, Instructor, (504) 527-6374, cnolan1@bellsouth.com

MAINE

Belfast	Sustainable Fitness, Beth Tracy, Instructor, 92 Main St., Belfast, ME 04915, (207) 338-2977
Camden	Maureen (Mo) Freeman, Instructor, 133 Washington St., Camden, ME 04843, (207) 230-0073
Cape Elizabeth	Nancy Eitner, Instructor, 10 Olde Fort Rd., Cape Elizabeth, ME 04107, (207) 799-4139
Rockland	Ily Shofestall, Brigitte Ziebell, Instructors, The Thorndike, 385 Main St., Rockland, ME 04841, (207) 596-6177

MASSACHUSETTS

Boston	Boston Bodyworks Studio, Kathryn Van Patten, Instructor, 12 Joy St., Boston, MA 02114, (617) 723-8090
Boston	Sarah Faller, Instructor, (617) 269-4300 x187
Boston	Progressive Bodyworks, Clare Dunphy-Foster, Cheryl Boyle Lathum, Vania Sacramento, Sarah Faller, Instructors, 441 Stuart St., Boston, MA 02116 (Back Bay), (617) 247-8090, strongbody@aol.com
Cambridge	Green Street Studios, Martha Mason, Lisa Silveria, Instructors, 185 Green St., Cambridge, MA 02139, (617) 491-2940
Gloucester	Joe Porcaro, Instructor, (978) 283-4531
Lenox	Uli Magel, Instructor, (888) 969-6668
Salem	Jimmy Raye, Instructor, 21 Salem St., Salem, MA 01970, (978) 741-1540
Stockbridge	Mathilde M. Klein, PT, Instructor, 21 South St., Box 1219, Stockbridge, MA 01262, (413) 298-3896
Wakefield	Flexfit Mind & Body Training Center, Carla Dunlap-Kann, Instructor, 607 North Ave., Soor 14, Wakefield, MA 01880, (781) 245-9143, coccobuns@carladunlap.com
Waltham	Fitness Finesse, Inc., Cheryl Lathum, Kathy Van Patten, Instructors, 411 Waverly Oaks Rd., #200, Waltham, MA 02452, (781) 736-0000

MARYLAND

Baltimore	Goucher College, Elizabeth Lowe Ahearn, Lynne Balliette, Linda Moxley, Instructors, 1021 Dulaney Valley Rd., Baltimore, MD 21204-2794, (410) 337-6399, Fax: (410) 337-6433, eahearn@goucher.edu
Frederick	Linda Rinier Moxley, Instructor, (301) 694-3015
Mount Rainier	Michael Rooks, Instructor, (301) 927-2134, rookery@worldnet.att.net

MICHIGAN

Detroit — Wayne State University, Theatre Dept., Nira Pullin, Instructor, 4841 Cass Ave., Suite 3225, Detroit, MI 48202, (313) 577-3508, (612) 672-6697 (for Univ. Theatre students only)

MISSOURI

Columbia — In Line Studio, Janice Dulak, Instructor, Stevens College, 1815 University Ave., Columbia, MO, (573) 442-2211 x4715

Kirkwood — Susan Bronstein, Instructor, 11830 Big Bend Rd., St. Louis, MO 63122, (314) 965-5672

St. Louis — Body and Mind Awareness, Caryle Flom, Instructor, (314) 721-8148, caryle_flom@email.com

(St. Louis Area) — Pam Moody, Instructor, 340 South Fillmore, Edwardsville, IL 62025, (618) 692-9763

NEW JERSEY

Absecon — Holly's Dance & Body Arts, Holly Bozzelli, Instructor, 119 Marin Dr., Absecon, NJ 08201, (609) 383-8822

Clifton — Karen Schoenberger, Instructor, (973) 779-7116, karsch@ix.netcom.com

Haledon — Julie LaRusso, Instructor, (973) 790-4243, gary-julie@worldnet.att.net

Hohokus — Body Tech, Kathryn Ross-Nash, Julie LaRusso, Instructors, 500 Barnett Pl., Hohokus, NJ 07423, (201) 444-6200, bodytech@pipeline.com

Kingston — Integrated Fitness, Donna C. Longo, Instructor, 4595 Route 27, Kingston, NJ 08528, POB 44, (609) 252-9229 and (609) 252-0997

Princeton — Anthony Rabara, Instructor, 377 Wall St., Princeton, NJ 08540, (609) 921-7990

Ridgewood — Arlene Dodd, Instructor, 75 Wilson St., Ridgewood, NJ 07450, (201) 455-3102

Tenafly — Jeannie Lee, Instructor, Tenafly, NJ 07670, (201) 568-0425

Titusville — Zane Rankin, Instructor, 50A River Dr., Titusville, NJ 08560, (609) 730-9544

Upper Montclair — The Movement Place, Holly Mensching, Karen Cooper, Sarah Ainsworth, Instructors, 48 Northview Ave., Upper Montclair, NJ 07043, (973) 746-2577

Waldwick — Pamela DeJohn, Instructor, 51 Waldwick Ave., Waldwick, NJ 07463, (201) 652-5986, pamdej@wordnet.att.net

Westmont — Donna M. Tambussi, Instructor, 20 Haddon Ave., Westmont, NJ 08108, (609) 869-3569

NEW MEXICO

Santa Fe — Kathleen Loeks, Instructor, 615 Calle de Leon, Santa Fe, NM 87505, (505) 984-2909, Fax: (505) 982-7411

Sante Fe — Stacy Weitzner, Instructor, (505) 988-4489, awgalt@worldnet.att.net

NEW YORK STATE

Albany — Body Wisdom, Ellen A. Weinstein, Owner/Instructor, 344 Fuller Rd., Albany, NY 12203, (518) 435-1064

Bedford	Vandy Lipman, Instructor, 66 Millbrook Rd., Bedford, NY 10506, (914) 234-6079
Briarcliff Manor	Saro Vanasup, Instructor, (914) 762-0040 (Westchester County)
Brooklyn	Jessica Fadem, Instructor, (718) 469-2265 (Park Slope)
Brooklyn	Body Tonic, Jennifer DeLuca, Instructor, 150 5th Ave., Brooklyn, NY 11215, (718) 622-2755
Brooklyn	Metta Coleman, PT, Instructor (Mount Sinai Hospital, NYC), Metira@aol.com
Brooklyn	Kara Springer, Instructor, 50 Clark St., Apt. 2C, Brooklyn, NY 11201, Kspringer@erols.com
Brooklyn	Rosanna Barberio, Instructor, (718) 246-2447
Cold Spring Harbor	Amy Wilson, Instructor, (516) 815-5505
Fishers Island	Susan Connelly, Instructor, P.O. Box 648, Fishers Island, NY 06390, (516) 788-7750
Glen Cove	Charmian's Center, Charmian Surface, Instructor, 13 Harbor Hill Rd., Glen Cove, NY 11542, (516) 671-0242
Great Neck	Fitness Studio at Marathon P. T., Doug Pollack, PT, Instructor/Owner, Ali Daniels, Ann Turner, Linda Figlia, Instructors, 330 Great Neck Rd., Great Neck, NY 11021 (Long Island), (516) 829-2938
Great Neck	Total Body Dynamics, Patricia O'Donnell, Instructor, (516) 944-0670
Greenlawn	Mary Lundo Studio, Mary Lundy, Instructor, 46 Fenwick St., Greenlawn, NY 11740, (516) 757-9050
Hastings-on-Hudson	Bodyscape, Kerry Donegan, Instructor, 5 Boulanger Plaza, (914) 478-2639
Huntington	Maggie Amrhein, Owner/Instructor, Teri Safaii, Amy Wilson, Instructors, 318 Main St., Huntington, NY 11743 (Long Island), (516) 421-1866
Irvington	Bella Flex Studio, Nancy Adler, Instructor, (914) 591-5690, adlern@email.msn.com
Katonah	Equipoise, Carol Dodge Baker, Vandy Lipman, Instructors, 113 Todd Rd., Katonah, NY 10536, (914) 232-3689, Fax: (914) 234-9289
Kingston	The Movement Center, Leah Chaback Feldman, Owner/Instructor/Teacher/Trainer, Elise Bacon, Beth Sullivan, Debra Noble, Instructors, 39 Broadway, Kingston, NY 12401, (914) 331-0986
Locust Valley	Fitness Studio at Marathon P. T., Doug Pollack, PT, Patricia O'Donnell, Ann Turner, Amy Wilson, Linda Figlia, Instructors, 22 Forest Ave., Locust Valley, NY 11560 (Long Island), (516) 671-8631
Locust Valley	Linda Figlia, Instructor, (718) 224-1695, Fra6301in@aol.com
Mount Kisco	The Art of Control, Simona Cipriani, Instructor/Owner, Tiziana Trovati, Megan Bridge, Instructors, 37 West Main St., Mount Kisco, NY 10569, (914) 242-0234
New Paltz	Elise Bacon, Instructor, 12 North Chestnut St., New Paltz, NY 12561, (914) 255-0559

For the most up-to-date information, please visit www.pilates-studio.com.

Port Washington	Susan Brilliant, Instructor, (516) 883-8298
Rhinebeck	Deni Bank, Instructor, Astor Square Mail, 88 Rt. 9N, Suite 20, Rhinebeck, NY 12572, (914) 876-5114
Riverdale	Kerry Donegan, Instructor, (718) 548-1175
Rye	Amy Aronson Studio, Instructor, 560 Polly Park Rd., Rye, NY 10580 (Westchester County), (914) 921-0522
St. Albans	Miyuki Kato, Instructor, 194-09 109th Ave., #1F, St. Albans, NY 11412, (718) 217-9814, miyuki.mclaurine@cwix.com
Saratoga Springs	Lisa Hoffmaster, PT, Instructor, 376 Broadway, Suite 5, Saratoga Springs, NY 02866, (518) 677-2557
Scarsdale	Center for Movement, Eleanor Jardim, Jean McCabe, Kathy Wolfe, Donna Krystofiak, Instructors, 846 Scarsdale Ave., Scarsdale, NY 10543, (914) 722-7646
Sleepy Hollow	Saro Vanasup, Instructor (Westchester County), (914) 524-9655
Southampton	Jeanette Davis, Instructor, 395 County Rd., #39A, Southampton, NY 11968, (516) 204-0122
Westhampton	Mary McGuire Wein, Instructor, (516) 325-3491
Woodbury	Tracy Greenfield, Instructor, (516) 319-4915
NEW YORK CITY: *(West Side)*	The Pilates Studio®, Sean P. Gallagher, PT, Director, Bob Liekens, Supervising Instructor/Teacher/Trainer, Sharon Henry, Kelly Hogan, Saro Vanasup, Stephanie Beatty, Ton Voogt, Michael Fritzke, Peter Fiasca, Sandra Zevner, Instructors, 2121 Broadway, Suite 201, New York, NY 10023 (between 74th and 75th Sts.), (212) 875-0189, Fax: (212) 769-2368
(West Side)	Cynthia Khoury, Instructor, 2130 Broadway, #1002, New York, NY 10023, (212) 787-0746
(West Side)	Mathilde M. Klein, PT, Instructor, 210 West 78th St., #3A, New York, NY 10023, (212) 595-3863
(West Side)	Reebok Sports Club, Monique Rhodriquez, Sharon Korty, Holly Cosner, Instructors, 160 Columbus Ave., New York, NY 10023, (212) 501-3685
(West Side)	Alicia Principe, Instructor, 210 West 101st St., New York, NY 10025, (212) 662-6025
(West Side)	Suzanne Jordan, Instructor, 55 West 111th St., New York, NY 10026, (212) 427-5238, szanjord@usa.com
(West Side)	Christina Richards, Instructor, (212) 362-8939
(West Side)	Kim Reis, Instructor, (212) 353-6813, Kikireis@aol.com
(West Side)	Monique Rhodriguez, Instructor, (212) 665-0575
(West Side)	Simone Cardoso, Instructor, (212) 582-9567
(West Side)	Junghee Kallander, Instructor, (212) 665-0575

(Midtown)	Drago's Gym, Romana Kryzanowska, Sari Pace, Master Teachers, Lori Oshansky, Jeanne Gross, Claude Assante, Instructors, 50 West 57th St., 6th Fl., New York, NY 10019, (212) 757-0724
(East Side)	The Pilates Studio® & Pilates®, Inc., Elyssa Rosenberg, Associate Director, Suzanne Jordan, Junghee Kallander, Stephanie Beatty, Instructors, 890 Broadway, 6th Fl., New York, NY 10003, (212) 358-7676, Fax: (212) 358-7678, (800) 474-5283 or (888) 474-5283
(East Side)	Makiko Oka, Instructor, East 60th St., (212) 308-0786, MakikoOka@aol.net
(East Side)	JRW Physical Therapy, Roberta Wein, PT, Instructor, Yohanna Ragins, Bernadette Ceravolo, Instructors, 60 East 56th St., 5th Fl., New York, NY 10022, (212) 688-6089
(East Side)	Cristina Gregon, Instructor, (212) 477-6288, cristi1009@aol.com
(East Side)	Pamela Pardi, Instructor, (212) 420-5925, ppardi5700@aol.com
(East Side, UN)	Christy Ann Brown, Instructor, (212) 973-0273
(Gramercy Park)	Susan Connelly, Instructor, (212) 228-1984
(Greenwich Village)	Diane Lam, Instructor, 526 Hudson St., #2F, New York, NY 10014, (212) 627-8605
(Greenwich Village)	Village Body Mechanics, Clain Dipalma, Instructor, New York, NY 10011, (212) 229-9369
(Greenwich Village)	Hanna Koren, Instructor, 46 Downing St., #5A, New York, NY 10014, (212) 645-0157
(NoHo)	re:AB, Brooke Siler, Owner/Instructor, Maria Hassabi, Daniela Ubide, Karin Weidner, Amy Wilson, Kara Springer, Elizabeth Stile, Instructors, 33 Bleecker St. at Mott St., Suite 2C, New York, NY 10012, (212) 420-9111, Fax: (212) 475-4103, reABNYC@aol.com, www.reabnyc.com
(SoHo)	Halle Markle, Instructor, 594 Broadway, #904, New York, NY 10012 (near Houston Street), (212) 431-8377
(SoHo)	Frances Craig, Instructor, (212) 925-4629, Fcraig@aol.com
(TriBeCa)	TriBeCa Bodyworks, Alycea Baylis, Instructor/Owner, Elizabeth Knock, Gina Papalia, Diane Lam, Angeline Shaka, Alison Thiern, Tizonia Trovati, Kathy Buccellato, Gabrielle Gregory, Rosanna Barberio, Instructors, 177 Duane St., New York, NY 10013, (212) 625-0777, Fax: (212) 625-0030, PilatesNYC@aol.com
(West Village)	James Duus, Instructor, 245 West 14th St., (212) 229-7674
NORTH CAROLINA	
Boone	Marianne Adams, Instructor, 665 Tarleton Circle, Boone, NC 28607, (828) 262-3028, Adamsm@appstate.edu
Chapel Hill	Celeste Neal Huntington, Instructor, 251 South Elliot Rd., Chapel Hill, NC 27514, (919) 929-1536
Swannanoa	Kathie Campbell, Instructor, 123 Long Beach Rd., Swannanoa, NC 28778, (828) 298-3623

Wilmington	The Studio, Ben Harris, Instructor, 7210 Wrightville Ave., Wilmington, NC 28403, (910) 509-1414, Fax: (910) 509-0116
OHIO	
Athens	The Body in Mind Studio, Marina Walchli, Leah Jean Rutkowski, Instructors, 9 Factory St., Athens, OH 45701, (740) 592-6090, Mwalchli:l@ohiou.edu
Athens	Leah Jean Rutkowski, Instructor, 11 Hocking St., Athens, OH 45701, (740) 589-6514, LR202595@oak.cats.ohiou.edu
Athens	Kris Kumfer, Instructor, Athens, OH 45701, (740) 597-6311
Cincinnati	BodyMind Balance, Inc., Jill Dema, Instructor, 3440 Edwards Rd., Cincinnati, OH 45208, (513) 871-6463
Ottawa	Jill Kuhlman, Instructor, (419) 532-3969, jk549196@oak.cat.ohiou.edu
OKLAHOMA	
Norman	Laura Wren, Instructor, 4017 Oxford Way Norman, OK, (405) 321-6171
OREGON	
Clackamas	Diane Caldwell, Instructor, (503) 698-4613, dcaldwell@imagina.com
Eugene	Susan Tate, Instructor, (541) 484-4011
Portland	Studio Adrienne, Adrienne Silveria, Instructor, Roxane Murata, Teacher/Trainer, 614 Southwest 11th Ave., Portland, OR 97205, (503) 227-1470, ELN/ro22@earthlink.net
Portland	Anne Egan, Instructor, 3424 Northeast 24th Ave., Portland, OR 97212, (503) 249-0823, Anne_Egan@Juno.com
PENNSYLVANIA	
Ambler	Peter Fiasca, Instructor, 208 Brookwood Dr., Ambler, PA 19002, (215) 205-8004, p.fiasca@worldnet.att.net
Chalfont	Zahra Nasser, Instructor, Chalfont, PA 18914, (215) 997-5640
Doylestown	Caroline Nolan Probst, Instructor, (215) 340-2222
Honesdale	Stone Gate Studios, Robin Dodson, Instructor, (570) 251-9408
Philadelphia	The Pilates Studio® @ the P.A. Ballet, June Hines, Megan Egan, Instructors, 1101 South Broad St., Philadelphia, PA 19147, (215) 551-7000, Fax: (215) 551-7224
Philadelphia	Alternative Health and Fitness Concepts, Janine Galati, Instructor, 2016 Walnut St., 2nd Fl., Philadelphia, PA 19103, (215) 567-4969
Philadelphia	Megan Bridge, Instructor, (215) 925-0244, meganbridge@falshcom.net
Pittsburgh	Dilla Mastrangelo, J. Christopher Potts, Instructors, 820 Maryland Ave., Pittsburgh, PA 15232, (412) 363-3426
Rydal	June Hines, Instructor, 1132 Dixon Lane, Rydal, PA 19046, (215) 576-8261
Titusville	The Rankin Studio, Sane Rankin, Instructor, 50A River Dr., Titusville, PA, (609) 730-9544
Wilkes Barre	Rosa Anne Serpico, Instructor, (570) 824-4391, rserp@prodigy.net

RHODE ISLAND

Barrington — Cassy DaSilva, Instructor, Barrington, RI 02806, (401) 247-2700, C1Angels@aol.com

East Greenwich — Body Mind Fitness, Inc., Deborah Montaquila, Instructor, 5 Division Street East, East Greenwich, RI 02818, (401) 885-2102

Johnston — Balanced Fitness, Linda Chavaree, Pam Turner, Instructors, 1665 Hartford Ave., #36, Johnston, RI 02919, (401) 528-1166

Providence — Body by Design, Inc., Catherine Cuzzone, Instructor, 126 Bayard St., Providence, RI 02906, (401) 421-7408

Warwick — P. Turner Studio at R.G.E., Pamela Turner, Instructor, 1775 Bald Hill Rd., Warwick, RI 02886, (401) 738-4401

SOUTH CAROLINA

Anderson — Edgar Tirado, Instructor, Camp Lou Ann, (864) 226-5439

Columbia — Ann Lore, Instructor, 128 Woodshore Ct., Columbia, SC 29223, (803) 788-7764, angelannsc@webtv.net

TENNESSEE

Franklin — Carrie Chrestman Leal, Instructor, (615) 579-6688

Memphis — Bodies in Motion, Sway Hodges, Instructor, 5111 Sanderlin Ave., Memphis, TN 38117, (901) 452-4976

Nashville — Greta Gryzwana Teague, Instructor, (615) 321-5100, epiphanydance@mindspring.com

Nashville — Willow Studio, Bambi Watt, Instructor, 5133 Harding Rd., Nashville, TN 37205, (615) 354-1955

Nashville — Spring Studio, Julie Kraft, Instructor, 2021 21st Ave. South, Suite 100 (old St. Bernards convent bldg.), Nashville, TN 37212, (615) 292-1930

Nashville — Bodies in Balance, Sylvia Gamonet, Greta Teague, Elizabeth McCoyd, Instructors, 1907-B Division St., 2nd Fl., Nashville, TN 37203, (615) 321-5100, Fax: (615) 321-5107

TEXAS

Austin — The Hills Fitness Center, Tracy Anderson, Instructor, 4615 Beecaves Rd., Austin, TX 78746, (512) 327-4881

Austin — Rachel Bhagat, Instructor, Rbhagat@hotmail.com

Austin — Vicki Hickerson, Instructor, Austin, TX 78731, (512) 452-0115, Fax: (512) 453-8619

Dallas — Body Proof Inc., Read Gendler, Instructor, 6706 Northaven Rd., Dallas, TX 75230, (214) 369-7273, Fax: (214) 369-7990

Galveston — Studio 424, Vicki Bolen. Instructor, 424 22nd St., Galveston, TX 77550, (409) 762-1399

UTAH

Salt Lake City — Katie Howard, Instructor, 2396 East Logan Way, Salt Lake City, UT 84108, (801) 582-4848

Salt Lake City	Body and Mind Studio, Claudia Flores, Instructor, 3300 South East, Suite 201, Salt Lake City, UT 84106, (801) 486-2660
VIRGINIA	
Arlington	Body Logic, Karen Garcia, Instructor, 3017 B Clarendon Blvd., Arlington, VA 22201, (703) 527-9626
Norfolk	Power House, Camilo Rodriguez, Todd Rosenlieb, Instructors, 134 West Olney Rd., Norfolk, VA 23510, (757) 622-4822
Richmond	4S Fitness, Inc., Jerry Weiss, Instructor, 2927A West Cary St., Richmond, VA 23221, (804) 355-5010
Virginia Beach	Studio P, Leslie Vise-Clark, Reid Strasma, Instructors, 4020 Bonney Rd., Suite 104, Virginia Beach, VA 23452, (757) 306-7077, Fax: (757) 306-7009
Virginia Beach	Axiom, Elyse Tapper Cardon, Instructor, 332 North, Great Neck Rd., Suite 105, Virginia Beach, VA, (757) 486-8665, Fax: (757) 486-8663, davelyse@aol.com
WASHINGTON, D.C.	Excel Movement Studio, Lesa McLaughlin, Theran MacNeil, Kerry Devivo, Christine Abbott, Instructors, 3407 8th St. NE, 2nd Fl., Washington, D.C. 20017, (202) 269-3020
	Fitness for Life, Brigitte Ziebell, Instructor, 1417 27th St. NW, Washington, D.C. 20007, (202) 338-6765
WASHINGTON	
Everett	Intrinsic Energy Studio, Bernadette Wilson, Instructor, 3426 Broadway, Suite 301A, Everett, WA 98201, (425) 252-8240
Kirkland	Atasha Avery, Instructor, 429 8th Ave., Kirkland, WA 98033, (206) 822-2448, atasha_a@hotmail.com
Seattle	The Pilates Studio® of Seattle & Capitol Hill Physical Therapy, Lauren Stephen, Director/Instructor, Lori Coleman Brown, PT, Director/Instructor, Dorothee Vandewalle, Teacher/Trainer, Chacha Guerrero, Bernadette Wilson, Danielle Stanley, Sachiko Glass, PT, Theresa Shape, Instructors, 413 Fairview Ave. North, Seattle, WA 98109, (206) 405-3560, Fax: (206) 405-3938
Seattle	Robert Leonard Spa, Chris Siris, Dorothee Vandewalle, Instructors, 2033 6th Ave., Seattle, WA 98121, (206) 441-9900, Agish@aol.com
Seattle	Jennifer Saltzman, Instructor, 915 East Pine St., #408, Seattle, WA 98112, (206) 726-1903
Seattle	Molly Ashenfelter, Instructor, 5747 37th Ave. NE, Seattle, WA 98105, (206) 522-6620
Shoreline	Peggy Z. Protz, Instructor, 102 North 171st St., Shoreline, WA 98133, (206) 533-0820, pez009@sttl.uswest.net
WISCONSIN	
Milwaukee	Body Mechanics Studio, Jennifer Goldbeck, Instructor, 807 North Jefferson, Milwaukee, WI 53202, (414) 224-8219

WYOMING	
Jackson	Sally Lynne Baker, Instructor, POB 10609, Jackson, WY 83002, (307) 734-8940, DLCrawf@aol.com
Teton Village	Interhealth Studio, Sally Baker, Instructor, P.O.B 10609, Jackson, WY 83002

International Certified Instructors

AUSTRALIA	
Surry Hills	The New York Studio of Pilates® of Australia, Cynthia Lochard, Director/Instructor, Roula Karitarzoglou, Edwina Ward, Instructors, Suite 12, Level 4146-56 Holt St., Surry Hills, 2010 Australia, Tel./Fax: 011-61296984689
Sydney	Powerhouse Personal Training, Gina Richter, Chris Lavelle, Instructors, Suite 2, 44 Smith St., Balmain (Sydney) NSW 2041, Tel.: 011-61298186234, Fax: 011-61298186235
Sydney	Paulina Quinteros, Instructor, Tel.: 011-61293577448, Pquinteros@hotmail.com
AUSTRIA	
Vienna	Performing Arts Studios Vienna, Gabriella Cimino, Instructor, Zieglergasse 7, 1070 Vienna, Austria, Tel./Fax: 011-4315235656
BERMUDA	
Warwick	Contrology! Bermuda Ltd., Sophia Cannonier, Instructor, 82 Southshore Rd., Nautilus House, Upper Level, Warwick, Bermuda, WK09, (441) 236-0336, Fax: (441) 236-7998
BRAZIL	
Puerto Allegre	Studio Balance, Allesandra Tegoni, Instructor, Av. Encantado, 410, Puerto Allegre-RS 90470-420, Tel.: 011-55513306346
São Paulo	The Pilates Studio®, Inelia Garcia, Director/Instructor, R. Estevan, Cecilia Delgado, R. Cincinato Braga, Instructors, 520, Bela Vista, São Paulo, Brazil, Tel./Fax: 011-55112848905
São Paulo	Bergson Queiroz, Instructor, Rua Herculano de Freitas, 237-Ap 187, São Paulo, SP Brazil 01308-020, Tel.: 011-55112345106
CANADA	
Calgary	Lynne Smith, Instructor, 924 17th Ave. SW, Calgary, Alberta, Canada T2TOA2, (403) 244-4448
London/Ontario	Michaela Sirbu, Instructor, London, Ontario, (519) 457-1371, mcs@lon.ionline.net
Montreal	Deja Griffith, Instructor, #414, 3025 Sherbrook Street West, Montreal, Quebec H3Z- I A I, (514) 989-8299
Winnipeg/Manitoba	Therese Desrosiers, Instructor, (204) 943-3614
CHILE	
Santiago	Marcela Ortiz De Zarate Broughton, Instructor, El Buen Camino 96808-B Penalolen, Santiago, Chile, Tel./Fax: 011-5622927485

For the most up-to-date information, please visit www.pilates-studio.com.

Santiago   Fransisca Molina, Instructor, Nueva Costanera 4076, Santiago, Chile, Tel./Fax: 011-5622287133

ENGLAND
Cornwall   Gayla Zukevich Stulce, Instructor, 6 Meadow Rise St., Columbus Major, Cornwall, UK TR96BL, Tel.: 011-441637881972, meadownse@aol.com

FRANCE
Marseille   Monica Germani, Instructor, 23 Rue de la Guadelupe, 13006 Marseille, France, Tel.: 011-91710303

Paris   Phillipe Taupin, Instructor, Le Centre du Marais, 39 Rue du Temple, 75006 Paris, France, Tel.: 011-33142729174, Fax: 011-33142729187

GERMANY
Berlin   Galina Rohleder, Instructor, Schluterstranbe 13, 10625 Berlin, Germany, Tel.: 011-49308231124

Frankfurt   Leigh Matthews, Mayra Rodriguez Matthews, Instructors, Hans-Thoma-Strasse 7 (H.h), 60596 Frankfurt, Tel.: 011-49696032156

Munich   Karin Weidner-Mubanda, Instructor, Tel.: 011-49899576841

Stuttgart   Davorka Kulenovic, Instructor, Sickstr. 32/70190, Stuttgart, Germany, Tel.: 011-497119239026

GREECE
Athens   Eugenia Papadopolou, Instructor, Corpus Ray, 4 Doxapatri St., 114 71 Athens, Greece, Tel.: 011-3013617290

Cyprus   Emily Papaloizou, Instructor, Tel.: 011-3575342582

ICELAND
Reykjavik   National School of Ballet in Iceland, Lisa S. T. Johannsson, Instructor, Engjateig 1, Reykjavik 105, Iceland, Tel.: 011-3545530660, Fax: 011-3545572948

JAPAN
Tokyo   University of the Sacred Heart, Yumi Takada, Instructor, Hiroo 4, Chome 3-1, Shibuya-Ku, Tokyo, Japan, Tel.: 011-81354853884

Tokyo   Makiko Oka, Instructor, 2-59-6 Ikebukuro, Toshima-Ku, Tokyo, Japan 171, Tel.: 011-8139846546

LATVIA
Riga   Studija Sports Pluss, Aija Peagle, Instructor, Blaumanu iela 5A, Riga, Latvia

NETHERLANDS
The Hague   Marjorie Oron, Jane Poerwoatmodjo, Instructors, Keizerstraat 167, 2584 BE The Hague, Netherlands, Tel.: 011-31703508684, Fax: 011-31703228285

Rosmalen   Manon Van Grunsven, Instructor, Jan Heymanslaan 1395246 BK Rosmalen, Tel.: 011-31736418956

PHILIPPINES
Manila   Cecile Sicangco lbarrola, Instructor, 227 Reposo St., Bel Air II, Makati, Manila, Philippines 1209, Tel.: 011-6328954465

PORTUGAL
Lisbon   Maria dos Anjos Machado, Rua de Angola, blc-6, 3-A, Encosta Da Carreira, 2750 Cas Cais, Portugal, Tel.: 011-35114865652

SPAIN
Barcelona   Estudio El Arte Del Control, Javier Perez Pont, Esperanza Aparicio Romero, Instructors, mazucase@teleline.es

Madrid   Estudio Lara, Lara Fermin, Instructor, C/Magallanes 28, 1 A, 28015 Madrid, Spain, Tel./Fax: 011-34915943863

Pilates at 82

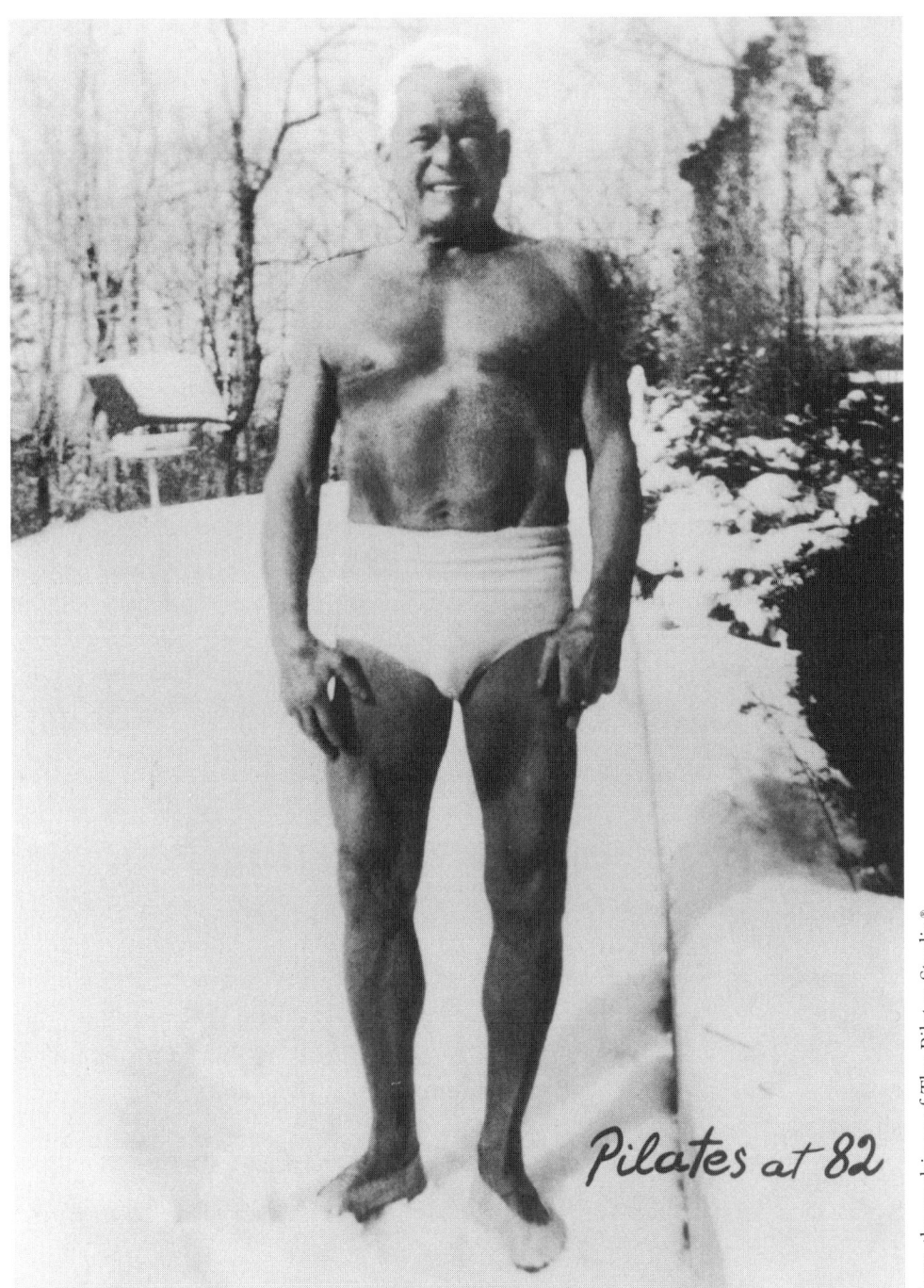

From the archives of The Pilates Studio®

Glossary

This is a very basic reference for the terms and names of muscles that are commonly used throughout this book. For more detailed information on the muscles, please consult an anatomical reference book.

MUSCLES

Hamstrings: The muscles/tendons that run up the back of the leg from your knee to your buttocks.

Quadriceps: A large group of muscles that run up the front of the thigh from the knee to the hip.

Obliques: The side muscles of the abdominals.

Triceps: The muscles that run up the back of the arm from the elbow to the shoulder.

Biceps: The muscles that run up the inside of the arm from the inside of the elbow to the armpit.

TERMS

Range of Motion: The scope of movement within which a muscle can comfortably be exercised.

Dynamic: The energetic output with which you perform the movements. In the matwork, dynamic is emphasized over speed. Your energy should match your level of control.

Momentum: The force with which you exert your movements. No exercises of the matwork should be performed by "throwing" your body around. The momentum for each movement should initiate in your center, or powerhouse, and remain controlled.

Articulation: In essence this is the act of segmenting, or putting space between the vertebrae, for example, as you roll up or down.

"Softening": The point at which your legs or arms can be straightened without locking your joint. (For example, "soft" knees are not locked or pushed into a hyperextended position.)

Hyperextension: The extension, or straightening, of body parts beyond their normal limits. (For example, when a leg "bows" backward at the knee joint, it is considered hyperextended.)

"Lengthening": The act of stretching or straightening without strain or tension in the muscle.

Pilates stance: The V position of the feet, heels together and toes a few inches apart, legs squeezing tightly together from the heels to the back of the upper inner thighs.

Powerhouse: The band of muscles that circle the body just under the beltline.

"Navel to Spine": The physical and mental act of connecting your abdominals to your spine to protect and engage the muscles of the powerhouse region.

Scoop: The act of pulling your navel down into your spine by contracting your abdominal muscles to create a concave, or "scooped," feeling in the belly.

About the Author

Brooke Siler is the owner of re:AB, the renowned studio for Pilates in NoHo, New York. Hailed as "trainer to the stars" by *Entertainment Tonight* and named as one of the top personal trainers in the country by *Vogue* magazine, Brooke is fast becoming one of the leading fitness gurus today.

Brooke was trained in the Pilates method of body conditioning by Romana Kryzanowska, the leading authority in the Pilates method alive today. Romana's thirty years studying and teaching directly under Joseph Pilates, plus an additional thirty years since, have earned her the title of the grand dame of Pilates. Brooke spent over six hundred hours under Romana's master tutelage and has since gained her own reputation as a highly respected teacher among those in her field.

After being certified by The Pilates Studio® in New York City, Brooke began privately training clients out of her apartment in Greenwich Village. Her reputation began to grow through word of mouth among her celebrity clientele, and it wasn't long before the press caught on. In 1997 Brooke accepted a partnership offer from her friend Michele Hicks, a top model and actress. Together they opened re:AB, a stylish, personable studio for one-on-one and group Pilates training sessions. Since re:AB's opening in June 1997, the studio has appeared on NBC News, NY1 News, E!, and VH-1, and has been featured in publications as diverse as *Elle, The New York Observer, Vogue, People, Harper's Bazaar,* and *Cosmopolitan.*

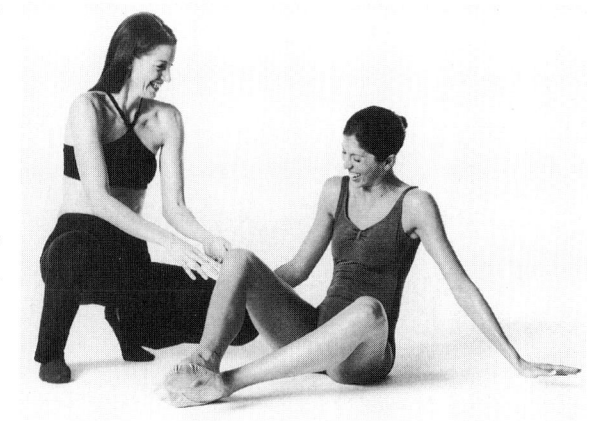